I0036505

Core versus Chore:
Using Human-Centered Design to Solve Burnout and Inefficiency in Healthcare

Grace E. Terrell, MD, MMM, CPE, FACP, FACPE

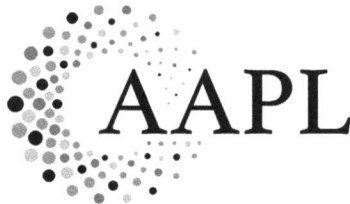

AAPL

Copyright © 2025 by **American Association for Physician Leadership**˙
Print: 978-1-960762-43-6
Ebook: 978-1-960762-44-3
Published by **American Association for Physician Leadership, Inc.**
PO Box 96503 | BMB 97493 | Washington, DC 20090-6503

Website: www.physicianleaders.org

All rights reserved. No part of this publication may be reproduced, stored in a
retrieval system, or transmitted in any form or by any means, electronic, mechanical,
photocopying, recording or otherwise, without prior written permission of the
American Association for Physician Leadership. Routine photocopying or electronic
distribution to others is a copyright violation.

AAPL books are available at special quantity discounts to use as premiums and sales
promotions, or for use in corporate training programs. For more information, please
write to Special Sales at journal@physicianleaders.org

This publication is designed to provide general information and is sold with the
understanding that neither the author nor the publisher is engaged in rendering legal,
accounting, ethical, or clinical advice. If legal or other expert advice is required, the
services of a competent professional person should be sought.

13   8 7 6 5 4 3 2 1

Copyedited, typeset, indexed, and printed in the United States of America

PUBLISHER
Nancy Collins

PRODUCTION MANAGER
Jennifer Weiss

DESIGN & LAYOUT
Carter Publishing Studio

COPYEDITOR
Patricia George

For my colleagues at IKS Health: Chalo!

TABLE OF CONTENTS

ABOUT THE AUTHOR

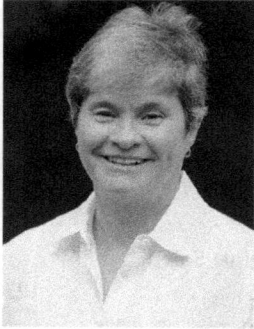

Grace E. Terrell, MD, MMM, FACP, FACPE, is a national thought leader in healthcare innovation and delivery system reform, and a serial entrepreneur in population health outcomes driven through patient care model design, clinical and information integration, and value-based payment models.

She is chief medical officer at IKS Health, an international healthcare company designing simple solutions for the complex problems in healthcare, using the "core vs. chore" framework. She has been a practicing general internist for more than thirty years. She has served as CEO of several companies, including Eventus WholeHealth, LLC., a company focused on providing holistic care to medically vulnerable adults and Cornerstone Health Care, one of the first medical groups to make the "move to value" by lowering the cost of care and improving its quality for the sickest, most vulnerable patients. She was the founding CEO of CHESS, a population health management company, and the former CEO of Envision Genomics, a company focused on the integration of precision medicine technology into population health frameworks for patients with rare and undiagnosed diseases.

Terrell has served as vice chair of the U.S. DHHS' Physician-Focused Payment Model Technical Advisory Committee, the chair of the board of the AMGA, and is a founding member of the Oliver Wyman Health Innovation Center. She is the author of several books, including *Value-Based Care and Payment Models, Reframing Contemporary Physician Leadership: We Started as Heroes,* and *Strategies for Recognizing and Eliminating Gender Bias for Healthcare Leaders.* She is currently executive in residence at Duke University School of Medicine's MMCi Program, a senior advisor for Oliver Wyman Health and Life Sciences consulting practice, and a member of the board of trustees of Guilford College.

INTRODUCTION: IMAGINE THE PRACTICE OF THE FUTURE

I am an optimist. I believe the medical practice of the future will be better than today's, and I am very invested in helping it be so. A few years ago, I formulated my personal mission statement: *I will use my talents, experiences, and scars and work with other people to radically improve healthcare.* Once I understood my professional mission, my career choices and work priorities became clear. Simply put, if what I am doing is not about radical improvement for physicians and their patients, then I need to change what I'm doing.

My current role, chief medical officer of IKS Healthcare, certainly fulfills that criterion. My company comprises more than 14,000 people, located in Australia, Canada, India, and the United States, who use our talents and technologies to eliminate many of the friction points that currently bog down the healthcare delivery system.

I wrote much of this book based on what I have learned working as part of this global talent juggernaut, which is focused on those "last mile" problems that must be solved before healthcare has a better, sustainable future.

One reason I am so passionate about improving healthcare is that I have witnessed both significant improvements and substantial diminishments over the course of my 40-year career in healthcare.

I started medical school in 1985, at the beginning of the AIDS epidemic, and I have seen firsthand a crisis of millions of people worldwide dying of a mysterious illness that attacked their immune system evolve into something that can be managed as a chronic disease and prevented altogether with appropriate public health and preventative strategies.

I have seen revolutionary improvements in the prevention and treatment of coronary artery disease and many cancers. Additionally, I have witnessed the development, in a matter of months, of the COVID-19 vaccines that lifted us out of our most recent pandemic.

But I have also seen the ongoing failure of our healthcare system to address cost, equity, and the prevention of chronic diseases. Like many of my fellow physicians, I despair at the ever-worsening administrative complexity we have to traverse every day to provide our patients with good care.

The other reason I am so passionate about improving healthcare is that my daughter, Robyn, has joined me in the medical profession, and I want her work environment and ability to provide care efficiently and effectively to be better than my own generation's experience.

Robyn Terrell Naron is a second-year pediatric resident at the University of North Carolina Health System. When she completes her training and enters practice in a few years, there should be far better workflows. These workflows will be built upon the tenets of human-centered design, incorporating the best of artificial intelligence technologies while maintaining the crucial healing role that exists in the doctor-patient relationship, itself embedded in millennia of human culture.

Robyn is a third-generation physician and, in fact, a third-generation female physician, as my mother-in-law, like me, was a general internist. I began my private practice in internal medicine in 1993 when I completed my training by joining my mother-in-law's and father-in-law's internal medicine practice. That was a wonderful opportunity for me in 1993, and permitted me the experience of practicing in an old-fashioned internal medicine practice where we saw our patients in the hospital, in the clinic, in the nursing home, and sometimes in their homes; did clinical documentation in paper charts; and performed a significant number of clinical procedures personally in both the hospital and clinic without consulting our specialist colleagues unless it was necessary.

Those days have long passed, and over the course of my career, the medical practice became part of Cornerstone Healthcare, where I served as chief executive officer, then part of the Wake Forest Health Network, then part of Atrium Health, and now Advocate Health, one of the largest healthcare delivery systems in the country. Along the way, the actual tasks of providing care got increasingly complicated, with complex electronic health records, patient portal messages that fill my inbox, ever-changing rules around prior authorization, medication reconciliation, and prescription refills, and "care gap" measures that do not actually measure outcomes, but, rather, identify missing process measure documentation.

All this can improve if we understand the true nature of the problem we are trying to resolve and use human-centered design to solve it. The problem is that chores have been added to dysfunctional clinical and administrative workflows in ways that lead to clinical and staff burnout, inefficient delivery of services, and higher costs.

This problem is not new. Several years ago, I was given a letter written to me when I was in medical school, which had never been mailed to me. It was written by my father-in-law, Dr. Eugene Terrell. He and my mother-in-law, Dr. Eldora Terrell, were internists who practiced medicine in High Point, North Carolina, from the 1950s to the 2000s.

Over the course of their careers, they saw medicine change in extraordinary ways. By 1987, when Eugene wrote this letter, the changes had taken the wind out of his sails. He never mailed it, but it eventually made its way into my hands. It offers a poignant, if cynical, view of the healthcare system that was beginning to break under regulatory and economic pressures:

Advice to my medical student daughter-in-law:

We were the original good guys. Keep the cost of medicine down, treat people based on need and not on ability to pay for medical care. We were frequently the last ones in the community to raise fees. One vivid memory stands out to haunt me. We ended our conversation at years end planning session with, "Let's wait until next year to raise fees, we can get by until then." My partner, board certified in internal medicine and neurology, kept his neurologic work up and consultation fees more in line with internal medicine fees. We kept a low-profile fee schedule but were able to raise fees when necessary. Needless to say, when Medicare froze our fees, we were already behind in our charges.

In spite of all this, our group gradually increased to a total of seven. Two neurologists, one pulmonary specialist, and four in general internal medicine. Our expenses rose dramatically along with our number of Medicare Patients. Collections fell in spite of two full time insurance clerks who stayed months behind trying to master paperwork, learning coding, follow-up checks, refiling claims, and experiencing long delays. In the midst of all this, our new business manager hired and sent to many courses in mastering the Medicare nightmare, suddenly died.

My world really started falling apart when we could not afford to rehire the last bright new young internist, and he left for greener pastures. After our fourth pay cut, the pulmonary specialist says, "I can do better than this on my own," and moved down the hall. The two neurologists with their higher fee profiles announced they were better off leaving.

The three of us left, all over 59 years of age, one over 70, and one a female tied down with her 92-year-old mother.

Can we start over? Can we avoid the mistakes and not go broke again? Maybe if I follow some of my advice.

My advice to our top-of-her-class, in Duke Medical School, daughter-in-law who wants to join us and whom we would dearly love to have:

1. Don't come back and join our group. You will be pegged into our low fee profiles, jeopardizing your ability to financially survive without the 80+ hour work weeks I know so well.

2. Don't go into general internal medicine. You don't get paid to spend long hours preventing diseases by teaching patients how to stop smoking, lose weight, eat properly, etc. Let them smoke. You get paid to treat their bronchitis and emphysema. Keep them fat. You get paid to treat their diabetes and hypertension. Don't worry about cholesterols. You get paid to treat angina and heart attacks. You lose money spending time keeping them healthy.

3. Do go into medical fields that do lots of procedures such as cardiology, neurology, gastroenterology, etc. I recently saw a bill to a patient in excess of $1000.00 for a less than one-hour EGD. I would have treated her for years for that kind of money. So, learn all the procedures you can. You get paid for these.

4. Don't go to post-graduate medical courses. Instead go to courses on how to do insurance and Medicare coding in order to get paid for the work you do. Learn to play the game with the yearly Medicare rule changes. (Last year's rules did not work either).

5. Charge all you can. Don't try to hold down cost. "They will get you," at the best you can do.

6. Don't take Medicare patients. They take longer, pay less and you lose money on everyone.

7. Don't get needed lab work on Medicare patients. You lose money every time.

8. Don't take these old nursing home patients. You don't get paid enough to treat them much less for all the time on the phone away from paying patients in the office or after hours at home.

9. Last of all, if you do get stuck with Medicare patients, get quick histories, do limited exams, get them in and out in a hurry. You can't

afford to treat 3-4 chronic diseases along with their acute illnesses. You don't get paid for all the time it takes.

I'm bitter, disappointed, depressed and tired but starting over. I love all these old people — they are appreciative and lovely to work with.

It's the system that got me.

Reading Eugene's words today, I see how much has changed — and how much hasn't. His experience of disillusionment and burnout is heartbreakingly familiar to many clinicians today, and his insights serve as a time capsule of the moment we began losing our way. Reading that letter makes me smile and makes me sad at the same time.

He was experiencing the first shock of the medical industrial complex, trying to manage the increasing costs of healthcare within the regulatory framework that we are still hurting from today. He was describing the personal burnout that we still experience from these same factors today, although he was feeling it even before the emergence of HCC risk adjustment coding, the electronic medical record, and the electronic inbox.

The letter makes me sad because he sounds so bitter, whereas my only experience with Eugene was as a kind, gentle man who never seemed to get angry at anything and never complained much at all. It makes me smile because I, of course, never heard this "advice" and would never have heeded it anyway.

I specialized in internal medicine, joined their practice, mostly see older patients, and have run one of the largest nursing home multispecialty practices in the country. Along the way, I've worked on fixing the payment system with value-based care policy work and primary care redesign, and am now the chief medical officer of a company whose entire business is built upon taking the burden of billing, coding, clinical documentation, inbox management, and other chores off the backs of clinicians. And my personal mission is to work in that company and with others to radically improve healthcare for Eugene's granddaughter, Robyn.

The medical specialty of pediatrics in which Robyn is specializing is currently in crisis, precipitating a shortage of pediatricians attributed to financial pressures from lower reimbursement, but also the "administrative burden of patient care oriented around the electronic medical record." Three pediatric professors from Robyn's program at the University of North Carolina at Chapel Hill declare, "the urgency of the moment means that children with all insurance types are currently having a hard time getting care, and it is going to get worse."[1]

It doesn't have to be this way. I imagine the practice of the future for her, where coding, clinical documentation, and medical billing are not tasks she has to worry about because these chores are done for her through a combination of advanced technology and a global human workforce. She is focused on the patient in front of her, is paid fairly for the work she does, and the work she does is the right work for the patient.

She has just-in-time information that is built to enhance the medical care she provides, not overwhelm her with the need to click endlessly in the infinitude of the electronic medical record. Gaps in care are unheard of because they are identified proactively and addressed accordingly. Her patients' needs are met promptly, based on best evidence for best outcomes, and she herself has a thriving medical career with no burnout.

The future I imagine for Robyn is absolutely achievable, but it requires a refocus at this critical juncture in the introduction of artificial intelligence into the healthcare delivery system. Healthcare has been called the only industry where technology has actually raised the cost of services. The information system capabilities of artificial intelligence technology can reverse that, provided we design it right. That starts with human-centered design principles.

The core theme of this book is that we can eliminate the chores that interfere with good care and professional satisfaction in the healthcare industry and design human-centered clinical and administrative workflows that eliminate burnout and inefficiency. The time is now to design a sustainable, satisfying physician profession for today and for the future. This future is not science fiction — it is within reach. But it demands intentional design, not just innovation. We must get rid of the chores that obscure the healing and reclaim the joy and purpose of being a physician.

PART ONE

Reimagine the Chores to Fortify the Core

Remembering the Core

I continue to practice medicine in an ambulatory clinic one weekend a month, seeing a group of patients who have been part of my internal medicine practice for over 30 years. One recent Saturday morning, the entire clinic was temporarily paralyzed by a health information technology glitch that was apparently affecting the entire six-state organization (40 hospitals and 1,400 care locations in the southeast United States) as a result of an "upgrade."

We found out that patients could not be registered to check in. The IT help desk in Charlotte assured us that they were working on it to the best of their ability. While we waited for the system to come back up, we brought the patients back and switched to paper documentation until we could transfer the information to the electronic health record later. We knew that our core mission was to take care of our patients, and this was the easiest way to keep them from waiting.

Unfortunately, not everyone that day had the same mindset. Several of my patients were fasting for lab work, so I provided hand-written prescriptions for the needed labs and sent them upstairs to the phlebotomy draw station so that they could get their labs drawn with the clinical information entered into the system later. I found out later that the team in the lab that morning sent the fasting patients home, telling them they could not draw their blood without the computer working. So, my patients, many of them elderly and frail, were sent back home without receiving their labs.

There is nothing impossible about drawing the bloodwork, carefully confirming the patients' names and dates of birth, and hand-labeling the vials of blood while waiting for the system to return to normal. It would have saved the affected patients a second day of fasting, a second day of having to travel back to the lab, and, in some cases, a second day that frail, elderly patients had to arrange for a family member or caregiver to accompany them to the lab.

Although one could argue that this experience demonstrates a lack of patient-centeredness in the care experience, I suspect it is instead an example of a more pervasive phenomenon: Many healthcare workers no longer distinguish between their core mission and the chores that make up the delivery of those services.

I believe the phlebotomists who turned away my patients did so with the understanding that their job was to use the lab information system they had been trained on to print labels and then draw the blood. When they ran into a snag with the health information system, they were paralyzed with respect to how to do their job. So, they did not actually do it.

Meanwhile, downstairs in the clinical setting, we were taking vital signs, talking to patients, examining patients, and determining medical assessments and plans. By distinguishing our core job — taking care of patients — from a chore associated with it — adequately documenting the clinical interaction in the electronic health record — we were able to satisfactorily perform our work with minimal disruption to patient flow. The medical assistant helping me that morning said, "Dr. Terrell, we're just old school — we know what to do!"

By referring to us as "old school," I believe the medical assistant understood that our core work is different from the tools we use to do that work, and therefore, we were able to innovate on the spot to keep the patients' needs and experience front and center. We carefully documented our clinical findings in the old-fashioned way — with pen and paper — and then later converted the paper to a proper electronic note.

Although the phlebotomy team could perhaps have argued that they would not draw blood safely without the lab information system up and running, I am not buying it. Careful attention to hand labeling with name and date of birth would resolve that, although it would have meant a little more work for them later on.

This isn't just about one clinic on one Saturday. Across the country, healthcare workers are conditioned to defer to systems of work rather than mission. When those systems fail, so does care. In a mission-focused environment, the core work ought to be easy to distinguish from the chores, to allow front-line workers to center their efforts on the critical work they do for patients. The distinction can also help resolve some of the wickedest problems we face in healthcare: excessive costs of providing services, clinician burnout, exorbitant levels of administrative burden, and poor patient experiences in the clinical setting.

I am the chief medical officer at IKS Healthcare because I believe separating the chores from a physician's core work is essential if we are to solve the ongoing problems of burnout, high cost, and poor clinical outcomes in our healthcare delivery system. IKS Health has spent the last 19 years designing solutions that reimagine the chores of healthcare as distinct problems to be solved within the clinical and administrative workflows.

We believe that care delivery models can be redesigned to manage the competing priorities that clinicians and their staff face. If a task does not have to be done by a physician, then it shouldn't be, and if it doesn't have to be done by the clinician's in-office staff, then it shouldn't be. Re-aligning tasks such that a technology-enabled global delivery team supports back-office extended care teams and in-clinic care teams can significantly reduce staff workload, improve efficiency, and reduce burnout.

Many colleagues are sounding the alarm about how the chores of healthcare are interfering with the ability to fulfill our professional core mission. Mary Tipton, MD, recently posted on LinkedIn about her decision to leave her primary care practice and join a concierge practice. She showed a screenshot of her assessment of a patient required by the "greedy vertically integrated" company she was leaving. The screenshot showed 22 separate diagnoses she was expected to assess, including seven different ways she was to code for diabetes, heart failure, COPD, obesity, and peripheral vascular disease. She wrote:[2]

> "THIS right here is why I can't continue this broken model. This is an actual (and typical) list of the codes I had to document for a recent visit for a Medicare Advantage patient. All the codes attested to in a 20-minute visit. 20 minutes with the patient and 60+ minutes later typing redundant and useless plans for each code. Who benefits here? Not the patient. Not the doctor. Only the greedy vertically companies that want the maximum risk score for their panel of patients and coerce physicians to cook the books for them in the name of accurate coding. It is wrong."

Tipton's strong reaction to coding diagnoses associated with risk-adjustment factor (RAF) scores leads her to nearly assert medical fraud in her frustration with the process. In fact, the whole purpose of risk adjustment coding is to identify patients who are at higher risk for adverse outcomes and develop models of care that better meet their needs and provide higher reimbursement due to their increased medical complexity.

Unfortunately, much of that purpose has been lost in the workflows that have defeated this physician, which likely were designed, as she said, to maximize reimbursement rather than maximize patient outcomes. Sadly, patients with these comorbidities are EXACTLY the patients who need good primary care. But the chores of clinical documentation, as experienced by Tipton, have driven someone who is likely a very good physician to a medical practice that is likely to have fewer such patients. Originally meant to drive care equity and resource allocation, RAF scoring has instead developed into a coding arms race, leaving physicians like Tipton feeling more like auditors than healers.

How in the world did we get to such a place where physicians, who have spent four years in college, four years in medical school, and then three years of training in internal medicine or family medicine, begin leaving clinical practice in droves due to the nature of the work they aspired to? Much of the problem, to my mind, has to do with how the nature of the job has changed. When I completed my training in 1993 and began my medical practice in internal medicine, I worked long, hard days, but the work was rewarding. I practiced medicine in the local hospital, just across the street from my medical office, saw patients in the office, and saw patients at a nursing home just a block away.

I began my day making rounds at the hospital at around 7 a.m., then arrived at my office at 8:30 a.m., and saw patients in the clinic until 4–5 p.m., when I returned to the hospital to check on my hospital patients once more. In both the hospital and office, I wrote my notes into a paper chart. My office nurse and I had a very efficient system of seeing patients with all sorts of clinical complexity.

A phone triage nurse handled most of the incoming calls from patients and the hospital and communicated back to the patients about tests and referrals. We could easily see 25 patients a day, and I could fill out a billing and coding front sheet in 30 seconds with the click of a pen. What we called the "orange sheet" kept a list of the patients' chronic problems, immunizations, medications, and health maintenance records, such as mammograms and pap smears.

The inefficiencies in the system were mostly related to inevitable medical emergencies, when my patients showed up at the emergency room in need of my immediate attention, calls from nursing staff at the hospital with questions about my inpatients that distracted me from my ambulatory patients, and a lack of integration of medical information. If I were on call for a doctor in another practice and one of his patients showed up for admission at the emergency room, I would have had no access to his outpatient records to help me evaluate the patient adequately.

Likewise, if I needed to admit a patient to the hospital from my practice in the middle of the day, all the patients on my office schedule that day would be inconvenienced with long waits, or the patient in the emergency department would have to wait for me to finish my office patients, which inevitably created conflict with the emergency department staff who wanted to "treat 'em and street 'em" or wanted me to admit them and get them out of the emergency department so a bed could open up for another patient.

Across America, the evolution of solutions to similar problems led to the development of what became known as the hospitalist movement and the advent of electronic medical records. With the debut of the hospitalist specialty, which specialized solely in the care of hospitalized patients, internal medicine physicians such as me ultimately had to choose whether to center their practice entirely on inpatients or entirely on outpatients. I had a hard time choosing and was literally the last internist in my local community to give up her inpatient practice.

This proved difficult, as I had to utilize our hospitalist group to cover for me when I was not available, and they did not find this satisfactory, as it decreased the volumes they wanted for their practice, and I was not a part of their integrated team. The hospitalist movement made hospital medicine more efficient at the unit level, with decreased lengths of stay compared to patients whose physicians were also seeing ambulatory patients and making admission and discharge decisions at the end of the day.

Theoretically, the decoupling of primary care and inpatient work with the rise of the hospitalist profession meant more patients could be seen and processed through the hospital, and more patients could be seen and processed through the ambulatory settings by bifurcating this work. In doing so, internists (and family physicians) who concentrated on ambulatory care became "PCPs" in the lingo and internists and family physicians who focused on inpatients became "hospitalists."

What it did for me on a personal level was remarkable. Suddenly, being on call was not so bad. The hospital did not call me all night long about patients with an acute change in conditions. Soon nurse-triage services reduced evening calls from ambulatory patients who learned to call for non-emergency problems during office hours or go to the emergency room if it was a true emergency.

The hospital payment system change called DRGs (Diagnostic-Related Groups) inevitably pushed the hospitalist care model because it became in the hospital's best interest to discharge patients earlier than they did when they were paid a per-day fee.

Medicare's Prospective Payment System, introduced in the 1980s, changed the inpatient payment model such that each hospital stay is assigned to a single DRG based on several factors, including primary diagnosis, secondary diagnoses, procedures performed, age and gender of the patient, and discharge status. Once assigned, the hospital receives a predefined payment amount for each case.

The DRG system incentivizes efficiency at the unit level of a single admission, because if hospitals control costs, they keep the difference between the DRG payment and the lower costs of delivering the services. This payment naturally encourages increased documentation and upcoding, as more complicated patients and services result in higher DRG payments.

The hospitalist movement arose from the DRG payment system, where cost pressures and shorter lengths of stay promoted its development. Beyond DRG alignment, hospitals favored the predictability and specialization of hospitalists, who allowed them to better manage throughput, meet quality metrics, and reduce legal exposure tied to outpatient-to-inpatient handoffs.

Lost in achieving the goal of increasing hospital efficiency has been the fragmentation of care between the inpatient and outpatient settings, inadequate care coordination at transitions of care, and shift-working physicians with short-term transitory relationships with the patients they care for.

Hospitalists have one of the highest rates of burnout among physicians, with more than 50% of hospitalists reporting at least one symptom of burnout.[3,4] Among workplace factors cited by hospitalists as contributing to burnout are many factors related to the "chores of their jobs," including:[5]

• Frequent pages or interruptions for non-emergent issues.
• Time spent on tasks related to case management or tasks below my practice.
• Time spent on tasks that are not reflective of working at the top of my license.
• Time spent on electronic medical records and documentation.
• Performing duties that should be completed by other personnel.
• Time spent in the electronic health record on documentation or reading notes.
• Time spent on orders in the electronic health record.

From a few hundred hospitalists at its inception in the late 1990s, the hospitalist specialty now comprises over 60,000 physicians, making it one of the largest medical specialties and one of the top 10 specialties with the highest burnout rates.[6]

Although the benefit for patients is shorter lengths of stay and more standardized and evidence-based care, they have not been all that thrilled with the changes brought about by the hospitalist movement. When the model changed in the 1990s, patients complained that they wanted "their doctor" to see them in the hospital, not some physician who was unfamiliar with them. And the shift-like nature of hospitalist work meant that often the discontinuity in the inpatient arena shifted from one physician to another every 12 hours and every three or four days.

These changes in who did what could not have happened without the simultaneous development of electronic health records, which allowed the viewing of patient medical records from one setting to another. No longer would a physician on call have to go by the office in the middle of the night to view the outpatient chart before going to the emergency room to admit a partner's patients with whom they were not familiar.

New chores started cropping up with the fragmentation inherent in all these changes. "Medication reconciliation" took up a whole new aspect of the office practice, for example. Back when I saw my own patients in the hospital, I knew what changes had been made to their medication because I, or the specialists I consulted, had made them. Now, with other people taking care of my patients at the hospital, I had to carefully review what changes were made and, on the fly, determine why.

Sometimes, meds were changed in the hospital for formulary reasons, like switching someone from Prilosec to Nexium due to a hospital contract. Sometimes medications were changed due to a temporary condition, like holding someone's hydrochlorothiazide when they came in with nausea and vomiting. Sometimes a medication was changed for no obvious reason, and I had to spend time searching for the medical records to determine what possibly could have led to the change.

When that practice of primary care medicine became separated from hospital work, medication reconciliation became a crucial new chore. Multiple studies have shown that poor medication reconciliation is responsible for up to 50% of medication errors during transition of care.[7,8]

Many physicians have similarly felt the burden of these changes. Dr. Ross L. Fisher mourns the ruination of primary care. He asserts that primary care outpatient general internal medicine is dead as a result of our current healthcare system that has "morphed into a bloated bureaucracy that has lost sight of what and who matters, blinded by self-serving fiscal dictates trenched in corporate greed and married to governmental incompetence."

He remembers being in clinical practice in the latter 1980s, when collegiality and collaboration among primary care physicians and specialists were the norm, and "managing patients in both the hospital and outpatient clinical settings allowed a steady continuity of care and growth of skills while better understanding your patient's illness and course." He explains:

> "General internists were physicians who were still valued and made a differ-ence in the clinical realm, not yet relegated to being unglorified triage nurses and secretarial data entry technicians upon whose talents were wasted. Medical records were simple and desired information was easy to find before copy-and-paste note bloat made EMR notes inaccurate and irrelevant. Documentation requirements did not intrude on life after work hours, and 'pajama time' wasn't a concept. Rigid nonsensical EMR limitations with end-less clicking and box checking that does not advance the well-being of the patients were inconceivable. Common sense and genuine fulfillment existed. There was very little 'moral injury', the lifeblood of today's 'burnout.'"[9]

Fisher plans to retire early and states he looks "grimly and pessimistically" at the future and sees "the inevitable collapse of our current healthcare system at a time when our country's needs will be at their greatest."

I am more optimistic. We have the opportunity to reconstruct a functional healthcare system by redirecting our clinicians back to what they are sup-posed to be doing and away from all these unnecessary chores that Fisher and I agree about: the relegation of primary care physicians to being "unglo-rified triage nurses and secretarial data entry technicians." As Fisher states, "it seems that primary care providers now only exist to document in the EMR that all preventive care and screenings are up to date, that their social determinants of health are documented (without any means to improve these), and refer out to specialists to provide care that was formerly managed by primary care physicians."[9]

We have an opportunity not just to undo the damage, but to design a future where clinicians focus on healing and support teams and systems handle the rest. The first step is remembering what the core really is.

CHAPTER 1

Unnecessary Chores

urnout doesn't stem from caring for patients; it stems from the unnecessary chores layered onto clinicians by poorly designed technology, excessive regulations, and fragmented workflows. Consequently, the actual nature of the work that clinicians and their teammates perform is changed and degraded. One study involving a community emergency department of physicians using electronic health records showed the mean percentage of time spent in direct contact with patients was 28%. The pooled weighted average time allocations were 44% on data entry, 28% in direct patient care, 12% reviewing test results and records, 13% in discussion with colleagues, and 3 % on other activities. The total mouse clicks per physician approached 4,000 during a busy 10-hour shift.[10]

A 2021 Mayo Clinic systematic review of over 5,000 studies found that physicians spend 37% of their workday interacting with EHRs; nurses spend 22%. The authors concluded that "EHRs have significant room for improvement in usability, functionality, and workflow optimization."[11]

Another study of 100 million patient encounters by 155,000 ambulatory medical subspecialists and primary care physicians in 417 health systems in 2020 found physicians spent an average of 16 minutes 14 seconds per encounter using EHRs, with chart review (33%), documentation (24%), and ordering (17%) functions accounting for most of the time, and the distribution of time spent by providers using EHRs varying greatly within specialty. While the proportion of time spent on various clinically focused functions was similar across specialties, 11% of EHR activity was after hours (see Table 1).

The use of electronic records for clinical documentation significantly increased the time spent on clinical documentation compared to paper charts. The apparent increase in clinical productivity associated with electronic documentation, however, primarily measured in RVUs, is likely the result of increased documentation, which permits higher billing codes. At the same time, increased delegation by clinicians to others is also independently associated with increased productivity.

TABLE 1. Time Spent per Encounter on Major Clinically Focused Electronic Health Record Functions

Function Category	Time (minutes)	% of Total Time
Chart review	322	33
Documentation	231	24
Orders	162	17
Message center	101	10
Patient discover	75	8
Other	47	5
Problem/diagnosis	17	2
Departure	9	1
History	7	1
Health maintenance	2	0
Alerts	1	0
Allergy	1	0

In a study of over 100 million ambulatory encounters, physicians spent more than half their EHR time on chart review, documentation, and ordering — activities that consume valuable time without always adding clinical value. Notably, 11% of EHR activity occurred after hours.

In other words, while EHRs may boost measured productivity in terms of RVUs, this is often achieved through expanded documentation and delegation, not increased meaningful care. One study found an 11% increase in RVUs when EHR tasks were delegated, suggesting that redistribution of these chores — not increasing clinical workload — drives the gains.[12]

The widespread adoption of electronic health records in medical care has led to increased documentation workload for physicians and decreased interaction with patients. Emerging evidence indicates that EHRs, as currently implemented, increase clerical workload and physician stress and interfere with direct physician-patient interaction, thereby diminishing professional satisfaction and contributing to professional burnout.

Prompted by these dismal facts, multiple solutions have been devised to solve for EHRs' limitations, including live scribes, virtual scribes, and now ambient listening artificial intelligence scribes. Substantial data indicate that these solutions reduce clinician burnout. Clinicians using medical scribes were associated with less self-reported after-hours EHR documentation, and physicians using scribes were associated with a higher likelihood of spending more than 75% of the visit interacting with the patient and less than 25% of the visit on a computer.[13]

The popularity of live, virtual, and AI-powered scribes underscores a deeper truth: Clinicians are eager to offload clerical chores. These tools don't just save time; they restore humanity to clinical encounters. Physicians who use scribes spend significantly more time face-to-face with patients and less time on screens.

For every hour of direct patient care, physicians spend nearly two additional hours on unpaid EHR and desk work. In Sinsky's study, physicians spent 27% of their total time on direct clinical face time with patients and 49.2% of their time on EHR and desk work. While in the examination room with patients, physicians spent 52.9% of the time on direct clinical facetime and 37% on EHR and desk work. In addition, physicians in the study reported one to two hours of after-hours work each night devoted mostly to EHR tasks.[14] Physicians report that administrative tasks required by EHRs could be performed more efficiently by clerks and transcriptionists.[15]

Electronic medical record systems improve the quality of patient care and decrease medical errors, but their financial cost-benefit is quite modest. The estimated net benefit from using an electronic medical record for a five-year period was $86,400 per provider, with the benefits accruing primarily from savings in drug expenditure, improved utilization of radiology tests, better capture of charges, and decreased billing errors.[16] EHRs have the potential to improve safety and reduce errors, but the real opportunity lies in redesigning *how* we use EHRs, not *whether* we use them.

In 2023, just as the pandemic was beginning to wane, the worsening problem of burnout, especially for primary care clinicians, was gaining attention at the policy level. The Agency for Healthcare Research and Quality (AHRQ), a U.S. federal agency that is responsible for improving the quality, safety, efficiency, and effectiveness of healthcare for all Americans, published its recommendations to mitigate clinician burnout. The agency suggested strategies to address the root causes of workplace stress, including:[17]

- Tactics to reduce the time physicians spend on clerical tasks like documentation, order entry, billing, and coding.
- Team-based care ideas to boost staff satisfaction, including effective use of huddles, pre-visit planning, and tactics to enhance workflows.
- Examples of work-life balance programs to help clinicians and staff restore professional and personal wellness.

- Strategies for building strong social connections within a practice, from peer support and coaching to buddy programs.
- Suggestions on reviewing incentives, payment, and other policies to ensure workplaces don't encourage overwork or unhealthy behaviors.

Notably, first on their list are tactics to reduce physician clerical chores.

CHAPTER 2

Information Chaos

I n addition to burdensome clerical tasks, clinicians today face a more subtle but equally harmful stressor: information chaos. When systems flood, fragment, or distort critical information, they create cognitive overload that can jeopardize both patient safety and physician performance. Managing information overload is a challenging task.

Electronic health records increase cognitive demands on physicians. Professor of medical physics R.J. Holden says, "According to the human factors paradigm for patient safety, health care work systems and innovation such as electronic medical records do not have direct effects on patient safety. Instead, their effects are contingent on how the clinical work system, whether computerized or not, shapes health care providers' performance of cognitive work processes."[18]

John W. Beasley and his colleagues coined the term "information chaos" to describe the overwhelming, disjointed, and error-prone information environments that characterize modern clinical work. They used a human factor engineering perspective to discuss the concept of information chaos in primary care and its implications for physician performance and patient safety.

Information chaos consists of various combinations *of information overload, information underload, information scatter, information conflict,* and *erroneous information* — all of which increase cognitive load, distract from patient care, and pose serious risks to safety. Beasley and colleagues provide a framework for understanding information chaos, its impact on physician mental workload and situation awareness, and its consequences.

Information chaos is a routine experience for primary care physicians. This phenomenon is not just inconvenient, annoying, and frustrating; it has implications for physician performance and patient safety.[19] In a survey of 52 physicians from 26 practices with commercial ambulatory care EMRs in place for at least two years, chief medical officers at four EMR vendors, and four national thought leaders, six major themes emerged:[20]

- EMRs facilitate within-office care coordination, chiefly by providing access to data during patient encounters and through electronic messaging.

- EMRs are less able to support coordination between clinicians and settings, in part due to their design and lack of standardization of key data elements required for information exchange.
- Managing information overflow from EMRs is a challenge for clinicians.
- Clinicians believe current EMRs cannot adequately capture the medical-decision-making process and future care plans to support coordination.
- Realizing EMRs' potential for facilitating coordination requires the evolution of practice operational processes.
- Current fee-for-service reimbursement encourages EMR use for documentation of billable events (office visits, procedures) and not for care coordination, which is not a billable activity.

Five sources of information chaos are:

1. Overload: Too much irrelevant or duplicative data (e.g., copy-pasted EHR notes).
2. Underload: Missing data (e.g., absent SNF discharge summaries).
3. Scatter: Data dispersed across systems, locations, or people.
4. Conflict: Contradictory data from different sources.
5. Error: Incorrect or outdated information that's propagated by EHR tools.

Table 2 outlines the five sources of information chaos and their implications for physicians.

Information chaos distracts clinicians from the primary work of the visit: care for the patient. The magnitude of information chaos on the quality of care is affected by several moderators. Interruptions can shift the physician's attention from the task in which she was originally engaged to the interrupting tasks. Once that shift in attention occurs, memory of the primary task begins to decay. Interruptions increase mental workload, reduce the ability to cope with information chaos, and thereby potentially impair performance.

Expertise can modulate information chaos. Physicians with more experience may have less mental workload than physicians with less expertise. Time availability to cope with information chaos is important for patient safety. Information chaos in a time-constrained environment can exacerbate physician performance.

So, one way of thinking about how to solve for the burnout, the "information chaos" with its "cognitive overload," is to understand how to reimagine

TABLE 2. Sources of Information Chaos

Sources of Information Chaos		Implications for Physicians
Information Overload	Occurs when there is too much data (written, verbal, nonverbal, memory) for the clinician to organize, synthesize, draw a conclusion from, or act.	EHRs encourage copying and pasting, which can add irrelevant information through the use of templates and the mixing of data needed for billing and legal protection with data needed for clinical care. Integration of multiple physicians' notes, laboratory and x-ray reports, and hospital and home health summaries in different formats can contribute to information overload.
Information Underload	Occurs when the necessary information is lacking.	For example, a physician does not have access to the skilled nursing facility (SNF) discharge summary,
Information Scatter	Occurs when needed information is located in multiple places.	In a primary care encounter, the physician may need to access information from an intake form, EHR, clinic consultant, or the patient's recollection.
Information Conflict	Occurs when the clinician is unable to determine which data is correct.	For example, the patient states they are taking one medicine, the physician thinks they are taking another, and the hospital discharge summary says something else entirely.
Erroneous Information	Occurs when the information is wrong.	For example, the patient states they are taking aspirin for pain, but they are actually taking acetaminophen. The copy and paste function of EHR exacerbates this by replicating the erroneous information in multiple notes and places.

clinical work and administrative work in organized systems of care. Although the concept of "practicing to the top of one's license" has been applied to think about expanding clinicians to get the physicians and other clinicians to do the work they were trained to do, rather than administrative and clinical tasks that others can do. In clinical documentation, for example, entering vital signs, asking screening questions for Medicare Wellness visits, and performing other information entry tasks can certainly be done by trained medical assistants rather than physicians, creating more efficient workflows.

To reduce information chaos, we must redesign workflows to route the right tasks to the right people using the right tools. Unfortunately, the electronic health record has been designed in large part around highly trained clinicians doing this work, including data entry. If it doesn't have to be done by a clinician, it shouldn't be. If it doesn't have to be done in person, it shouldn't be. However, more often than not, the EHR technology was designed in such a way as to force those workflows on the clinicians.

Once the tasks of providing care are broken into constituent components, new ways of imagining healthcare work are possible. On the clinical side, a clinician can be supported by an in-clinic team, an extended care team outside the office, and even a tech-enabled globalized delivery team. Pre-visit summaries prepared by extended care teams, remote scribes documenting encounters, and AI-driven inbox triage are just a few examples of redistributing cognitive work away from frontline clinicians.

Breaking down the constituent parts of care delivery — before visits, during visits, after visits, in between visits, and in acute care settings — and solving for what parts can be redesigned for more cost-effective and more efficient care is crucial in innovating our way out of the burnout trap. Global clinical teams can review charts and tee up pre-visit summaries for busy clinicians so the clinicians have just the right information at the right time and do not have to spend their time combing through the EHR or chasing down reports from SNFs and hospitals.

Clinical scribes can write their notes and enter orders remotely. Billing and coding can be done with a global human workforce. And redesigned technology can take the burden of prior authorizations and inbox management off the plates of busy clinicians and their office staff.

Time pressures and noncognitive clinical tasks such as data entry, coding, and clinical documentation all contribute to the cognitive burden of information chaos. Information chaos can be combated with a focus on several critical factors:

- **Interoperability** between various data systems.
- **Information filtering and summarization** using artificial intelligence or summarization to distill key facts.
- **Human-centered design** that makes interactions more intuitive and decision-friendly.
- **Training and workflow redesign** to equip clinicians and their staff to manage complex information environments.

Focusing on these four critical factors can mitigate information chaos.

A bold example of this principle in action comes from Jackson Steinkamp and colleagues, who designed an EMR to eliminate one of the biggest contributors to information chaos: the clinical note itself. In 2021, Steinkamp and his colleagues published a paper on a fully collaborative noteless electronic medical record that they designed to minimize information chaos. They built a medical documentation system that does not use notes and instead treats the chart as a single, dynamically updating, and fully collaborative workspace. All information is organized by clinical topic or problem, and version history functionality enables granular tracking of changes over time.

The system is highly customizable to individual workflows, enabling each user to decide which data should be structured and which should be unstructured, allowing individuals to leverage the advantages of structured templating and clinical decision support.

Their new electronic health record was built on two design principles: (1) designing to minimize information chaos and (2) designing with baked-in clinical decision support. Information chaos was reduced by starting with the default assumption that information will remain the same over time, and information that changes is the exception. Therefore, a patient's accumulated past medical history will rarely be changed once recorded, and many aspects of a patient's current medical state will remain the same between two consecutive clinical notes. This means that the system's interactions were designed around small-scale changes of individual data elements without requiring redocumentation of the remainder of the unchanged data.[21]

The redesigned EHR was built around four design principles:

1. One shared workspace.
2. Dynamic updating by problem/topic.
3. Avoidance of note duplication.
4. Customization by role/user.

Steinkamp and colleagues' thinking is exactly the type of thinking that will get us to the improved state of healthcare delivery we aspire to. Their objective was to demonstrate the feasibility of building an EMR that does not use notes as the core organization unit for unstructured data, and that is designed specifically to disincentivize information duplication and information scattering that make up a large portion of information chaos in the clinician's day-to-day activities. Their system rethinks the structure of digital documentation itself, offering a glimpse of what's possible when design starts with clinical cognitive needs, not billing checklists.

A systematic review of the influence of electronic health record design on usability and medication safety published in January 2025 concluded that EHR systems that prioritized seven broad design themes were associated with higher reported usability and enhanced medication safety: search-ability, automation, customization, data entry, workflow, user guidance, and interoperability. The authors conclude that future EHR evaluations should be performed throughout the design process, and consensus building is nec-essary regarding what exactly constitutes a design element within the EHR context.[22]

Solving information chaos isn't about working harder; it's about working smarter, clarifying which workflows serve the mission and which ones are distractions. When clinicians can focus on diagnosis, decision-making, and healing, while support systems handle the rest, burnout declines, and quality of care improves. That's the promise of separating core from chore.

CHAPTER 3

Requirements for Fixing Healthcare Delivery

Fixing healthcare isn't just about payment reform or new technology — it's about redesigning the work itself. Broken administrative, clinical, and value-based care workflows drive burnout, inefficiency, and poor outcomes. We need a practical framework to untangle and rebuild them. It's one thing to declare that the critical core mission for physicians is to help patients and that this should be differentiated from the chores of providing that care. It's another thing to understand how to separate those things practically in order to make the mission-critical work as efficient and meaningful as possible.

Clinicians sometimes fail to distinguish between the work that is core to their professional training and that which has become increasingly burdensome chores. One easy way to do this is to ask a physician how much they enjoy documenting in the clinical chart, approving prior authorizations, coding evaluation-and-management services, and signing off on physician therapy orders. They will likely look at you as if you are crazy, begin complaining about their ever-increasing degree of burden these activities occupy in their workday, or just shrug and say that they are the necessary tasks that must get done in order to take care of patients.

Ask the same physician to describe what they like about their work, and you will likely get a description of a patient interaction in which they diagnosed an unusual condition, a statement about the deep, meaningful relationships they have experienced with patients they have helped, or, perhaps, satisfaction in mastery-level skills in a complex surgical procedure or other clinical expertise. These are the aspects of clinical work for which physicians have trained, but that occur within an environment where complex tasks are performed in order to accomplish this work and get paid for it.

Workflow is a sequence of steps, from a beginning to an ending, that delivers a service, produces and/or delivers a product, or processes information. The concept of workflows has a long history that spans several disciplines, including manufacturing, industrial engineering, and computer science. The idea of a workflow has evolved from manual labor optimization, not automated digital processes, but the core principle of improving task flow and efficiency has remained constant. Most physicians are not trained industrial engineers with experience in workflow mapping or redesigning business processes, but having a basic understanding of how clinical work is organized is useful in designing more efficient and sustainable healthcare environments.

Frank and Lillian Gilbreth were industrial engineers who created the first process charts using symbolic representation over a hundred years ago. Workflow chart symbols were standardized in 1985 with the International Standard for Process Documentation (ISO 5807). The modern workflow symbols indicate such factors as tasks, decision points, starts and ends, and inputs and outputs. These concepts are then built into a basic diagram of how a work process is organized (see Figure 1).

In healthcare, a workflow is a repeatable sequence of clinical or administrative steps that leads to a specific patient or practice outcome, such as registering a patient, performing a well-child visit, or submitting a claim

In an ambulatory medical practice, there are workflows for:

- Answering phones.
- Making appointments.
- Responding to inbox messages.
- Making and coordinating referrals, completing patient work-ups.
- Educating patients and their families.
- Planning patient visits.
- Consulting with other specialists.
- Registering patients.
- Entering vital signs.
- Identifying chronic and preventative care needs.
- Ordering labs and imaging studies.
- Arranging consults and therapies.
- Refilling prescriptions.
- Evaluating test results.
- Communicating test results.
- Billing for provided services.
- Administering immunizations or drugs.
- Performing procedures.
- Identifying gaps in care and opportunities to improve quality.

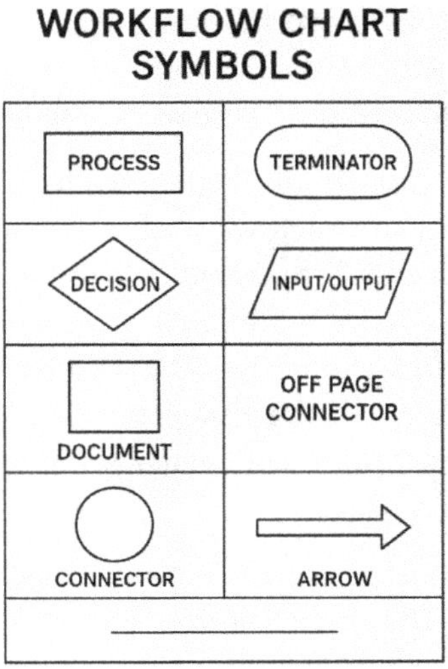

WORKFLOW CHART SYMBOLS

Figure 1. Workflow Chart Symbols

Different types of patient groups may require specific clinical workflows for preventative care, acute problems, chronic conditions, complex care needs, mental health, well-child visits, pregnancy, palliative/end-of-life, and post-procedure follow-up. By understanding these clinical workflows, one can redesign those that are inefficient and unnecessarily burdensome for physicians and their clinical staff.[23]

Workflow redesign isn't just a management technique; it's a strategy to restore purpose, reduce burnout, and improve patient care. In the current healthcare environment, the maddeningly complex interaction of clinical practice workflows, administrative workflows, and the change management necessary to adapt to new business models, such as value-based care, is converging into massive, stressful forces that strain the traditional practice of medicine.

These forces interact in the delivery system environment, contending with increased regulatory compliance expectations, inefficient bureaucratic payment processes required from a myriad of third-party payers, and ongoing shortages of physicians, clinical and clerical staff, as well as ongoing downward pressures on revenue.

By breaking down these complex problems into three distinct and critical workflows, clinicians can begin to resolve the complexity. They should ask three questions:

1. How should I solve clinical workflow needs?
2. How should I solve administrative workflow needs?
3. How should I solve value-based care workflow needs?

Each of these workflow needs is interdependent on the others in the complex healthcare environments in which we work. Clinical workflows encompass everything from well-visits to the screenings, labs, and follow-ups associated with the visits. Administrative workflows may include processing referrals and refilling prescriptions. An example of a value-based care workflow is identifying gaps in the care of a diabetic patient under a shared savings contract. Understanding these interdependencies and how to navigate them is a crucial part of reducing burnout.

National policy leaders are paying increasing attention to the importance of redesigning workflow. The American Medical Association added a Workflow Redesign Toolkit to its Steps Forward program. This structured framework is built upon stopping unnecessary work, sharing necessary tasks with a broader team, and gaining leadership support.[24] The National Academy of Medicine has amassed a compendium of key resources for improving clinician wellbeing that includes assessments of workplace efficiency.[25]

CHAPTER 4

More Efficient and Effective Clinical Workflows

Clinical workflows should make it easier, not harder, for clinicians to care for patients. Yet in most health systems today, clinicians are inundated with tasks that have little to do with medical decision-making. Reclaiming efficiency requires a radical redesign of who does what, where, and why.

Several basic principles can help build streamlined solutions, all based on our core-versus-chore test as a standalone principle:

- If it doesn't have to be done by a clinician, it shouldn't be.
- If it doesn't have to be done by a nurse, it shouldn't be.
- If it doesn't have to be done in the exam room, it shouldn't be.
- If it doesn't have to be done in the clinical office, it shouldn't be.
- If it doesn't have to be done inside the healthcare organization, sometimes it shouldn't be.

When workflows are rebuilt with these principles in mind, clinical teams can practice at the top of their license and reclaim time for patient care.

By distinguishing between the true core work of the clinical team and the chores that make up the workflow, breaking up the jobs into their constituent parts, we can devise new workflows that are more efficient, scalable, and more professionally rewarding for the core clinical team. Moreover, "practicing at the top of one's license" becomes possible again.

Unnecessary inbox messages are not just irritating — they are a form of unfiltered cognitive load. When physicians receive thousands of low-value alerts, the signal gets drowned out by the noise.

In the past few years, the electronic health record that my medical practice uses was built to facilitate the multistate, multihospital health system we are part of. It was not designed, however, around the principles of core versus chore. Ninety percent of the inbox messages I receive could and should be handled by someone else. Many of the notifications I receive are unnecessary, and new ones pop up every day.

Recently, I began receiving notifications when my pacemaker patients have their pacemakers interrogated by the cardiology practice. Now, I am not in any way managing their pacemakers and do not need notification that their pacemakers have been routinely interrogated and are fine. I should be notified if the patient is having a medical problem that I am managing that could be impacted by a dysfunctional pacemaker, but that would be rare and likely could be determined at the point of care when I saw the patient.

I presume someone in the organization determined that all primary care physicians would get copied on pacemaker interrogation reports. That's hundreds of unnecessary inbox messages for physicians throughout the organization.

Another example is the organization's recent decision that certified medical assistants would not be allowed to enter orders for physicians that physicians would then sign off on. Up until this recent policy change, I would enter into a lab report result note if I wanted additional studies, medications, or referrals done. My medical assistant would enter these orders, and I would review and sign off on them. Now, I have to enter information on the result note, and then spend a considerable amount of time entering the orders myself. I am serving what used to be a clerical entry role.

In preparing for a clinical interaction with my patients, I must review multiple fields in the electronic health record to determine what has occurred with my patients since the last clinical interaction, including lab results, imaging studies, specialist consultations, and telephone interactions. I may have to click on another part of the chart to review medical records from outside our health system. I will be asked to evaluate and assess clinical conditions that may increase coding value for patients in risk contracts, or explain that I am not going to do so at this visit.

I will be provided with a list of potential gaps in care and then have to search the chart to determine whether these gaps are real, such as when the patient has already had a DEXA scan to assess bone density, but the results are not captured in a discrete data field. I perform a diabetic foot exam on my diabetic patients with each visit, but unless I click through multiple discrete data fields to record it, it is not captured by the electronic health record and will be recorded as a quality gap.

While the inefficiency of navigating the EHR is one component of workflow burden, another is the limitations of current technology tools, such as ambient scribes. While ambient AI scribes can reduce typing time, they introduce new burdens: Clinicians must carefully review notes for hallucinations (fabricated or inaccurate AI-generated content), correct errors, and still complete documentation, orders, and billing codes. The ambient listening scribing tool provided for my use will capture a lot of detail of the conversation I had with the patient, but I will need to read the transcript carefully to check for hallucinations and edit inaccurate information, then provide clinical documentation for my evaluation and plan, enter orders, and, finally, accurately code the note. None of this is efficient.

CHAPTER 5

More Efficient and Effective Administrative Workflows

Within the context of administrative workflows, the same principles applied to clinical workflows hold true: If a task doesn't require the expertise of a physician or in-office clinical staff, it should be delegated or streamlined.

Consider the numerous steps required for a physician to be reimbursed for a single medical service. Before a patient even enters the clinic, the physician must be credentialed by the health insurer that covers the patient's care or must determine how to receive direct payment. Credentialing itself is a bureaucratic, often lengthy process involving submission of medical education and training records, licensure, board certifications, references, hospital privileges, and, in some cases, criminal background checks. This process may require review by the health plan's credentialing committee, which can take anywhere from three to six months, delaying revenue generation and limiting patient access to care in the meantime.

Once a patient initiates care — either directly or via referral — several steps follow:

- **Pre-visit tasks** such as eligibility and benefits verification (EBV), upfront co-pay or deductible determination, and medical records collection from outside facilities or providers.
- **Patient intake**, including questionnaires regarding past medical history, medication use, and allergies — all before any clinical evaluation begins.

Following the visit, the workflow becomes even more complex:

- **Documentation** must meet accuracy and compliance standards.
- **Coding** must align with billing rules and accurately reflect services rendered.
- **Orders** for labs, imaging, medications, or referrals must be entered into the EHR and executed — often requiring prior authorizations from insurers.

- **Claims** are submitted through electronic systems and typically processed through a *claims scrubber*, software that checks for formatting errors and compliance to prevent denials.

Even when these steps are completed correctly, payment is not guaranteed. Payers may deny claims for a host of reasons:

- Patient ineligibility (e.g., lapsed coverage).
- Incomplete or inaccurate documentation.
- Coding discrepancies.
- Payer-specific rule changes (which often vary not only between insurers but year to year within the same plan).

When claims are denied, the burden falls on the practice to troubleshoot, correct, and resubmit the labor-intensive claim process, requiring dedicated billing expertise. Alternatively, costs may be passed on to the patient, or the provider may write off the loss entirely.

This laborious sequence illustrates why administrative workflows are a significant contributor to physician and staff burnout and inefficiency. They require time, expertise, and resources that could otherwise be spent on patient care. Many of these tasks can be outsourced, automated, or redesigned through workflow innovation and team-based delegation. Global back-office support services, AI-enabled coding tools, and centralized credentialing systems are just a few of the available solutions that could reduce these burdens.

CHAPTER 6

More Efficient and Effective Value-Based Care Workflows

V alue-based care introduces a distinct layer of workflow complexity. It requires not only clinical expertise, but also data integration, care coordination, and financial stewardship within new and evolving payment models. Unlike fee-for-service systems that reward volume, value-based care incentivizes outcomes — meaning the entire delivery model must adapt to prioritize proactive, preventive, and personalized care.

At the core of value-based care is care model redesign, which must align with patients' clinical risks and social needs. This begins with identifying high-risk cohorts — patients with multiple chronic conditions, adverse social determinants of health (SDOH), rare diseases, or high-cost utilization patterns. Stratifying these populations requires synthesizing data from disparate sources:

- Electronic health records (EHRs).
- Insurance claims.
- Pharmacy data.
- SDOH indicators like ZIP code, food insecurity, or housing status.

These data must be unified into actionable insights that enable care teams to develop effective outreach and treatment plans. Yet, many EHRs are not optimized for this purpose, and clinical workflows built for fee-for-service models are poorly equipped to handle population-level interventions like:

- Remote patient monitoring.
- Care gap closure campaigns.
- Proactive medication management.
- Social services navigation.
- Multidisciplinary case reviews.

To add complexity, the payment side of value-based care involves managing a spectrum of financial models:

- Pay-for-performance.
- Shared savings arrangements.
- Upside/downside risk contracts.
- Full capitation or global budgets.

Each payment model requires its own set of administrative workflows for tracking performance metrics, managing budgets, forecasting utilization, and coordinating incentives across teams. Traditional practice management systems are rarely designed to support these financial flows, often requiring parallel tools or external vendors to support actuarial modeling, risk adjustment coding, and quality score optimization.

As with clinical and administrative workflows, the key to successful value-based care is task differentiation — high-level clinical decision-making. But the work of collecting risk data, flagging care gaps, coordinating social services, and documenting quality measures can and should be delegated to other trained team members or supported by specialized external teams.

Redesigning workflows around value-based care is not just a technical adjustment; it is a strategic realignment of mission and capacity. It allows physicians to return to their core professional purpose: healing and human connection. The rest — the data capture, metric tracking, and risk modeling — can and should be managed as distinct chores, not core functions.

CHAPTER 7

The Important Difference Between Professionalism and "Top of License"

n healthcare, as in broader culture, buzzwords come and go. "Groovy" became "cool," and now "rizz" rules the day. In the early 2000s, one such term entered healthcare's lexicon with striking momentum: "top of license." This phrase refers to the idea that every healthcare professional should perform only those tasks that align with the highest level of their training and credentials. Nurses should do nursing work, not clerical work. Physicians should focus on diagnosing and treating, not refilling routine medications or reviewing normal mammogram reports. The concept gained traction alongside the rise of team-based care and the early stages of value-based care.

As clinical complexity increased and staffing shortages worsened, optimizing team members' time became essential. In theory, this model supports both efficiency and quality by ensuring everyone practices to their full capacity, optimizing workforce potential, and improving patient outcomes.

The idea is that healthcare professionals can provide improved care as part of teams where nurses, advanced practice providers, and other allied health workers perform tasks that align with their training and expertise, leading to better teamwork and allowing physicians to focus on more complex cases. By ensuring that each team member operates at the top of their license, healthcare organizations can optimize their workforce to maximize resources in settings where staffing shortages and increased patient loads are prevalent.

As the concept of value-based care began to permeate the healthcare industry vernacular, it became apparent that the one-to-one relationship between a physician and a patient was, in and of itself, inadequate to deliver the highest quality care. The inefficiency of everything being pushed to the physician, despite the fact that the physician had a support staff to do much of the nonclinical work, was increasingly apparent.

In the fee-for-service payment model, the efficiency is at the individual provider unit level, whether considering an ambulatory visit, an imaging study, or a surgical procedure. You do as many units of the service as you can do, as efficiently as possible, and take home the difference between revenue per unit service and expense per unit service as your profit. Such a payment system rewards efficiency at the unit level and encourages investment in capacity. It does not reward high quality unless that leads to an increase in volume or a decrease in liability risk.

As medical services have become increasingly complex, having a physician at the top of a hierarchical pyramid is not always the most effective structure with respect to quality and outcomes. The healthcare industry has recognized the need to be redesigned for efficiency at the population level, in addition to providing highly efficient care at the service unit level.

The role of the surgeon is crucial in the operating room, but she is part of a broader team that includes the anesthesiologist, the certified nurse anesthetist, the scrub tech, the circulating nurse, the physician assistant, the scrub nurse, and the surgical assistant. Likewise, in an ambulatory setting, a clinical team that includes physicians, advanced practice providers, registered nurses, medical assistants, nurse triage, front desk staff, and clinical coordinators working together can provide much better care in a team matrix than in a hierarchical structure.

In team-based care, the responsibilities of individual team members should be defined to encompass their entire capabilities. Nurses should do nursing work, not medical assistant work. Physicians should do physician work, not medical assistant work. Yet in many health systems, the actual workflow is not conducive to this efficient use of teams. The physician's inbox on the EHR, for example, often contains a waste basket of items that do not require a physician's training to address.

Practicing at the top of one's license is based on the idea that the most efficient teams are built with each person doing the work they are most qualified to do. However, a critical distinction is often overlooked: *"top of license" is a productivity framework; professionalism is a moral and ethical compass.* The former organizes workflow; the latter defines purpose.

Professionalism in medicine is rooted in compassionate care, lifelong learning, clinical excellence, and an unwavering commitment to patients. It places the patient's welfare above self-interest. Practicing at the top of one's license should be an *expression* of professionalism. Unfortunately, it too often becomes a substitute, reduced to a labor division without reflection on meaning, responsibility, or human connection.

As healthcare delivery evolves, we are reminded that complex, high-quality care is rarely delivered alone. Modern healthcare must be structured around interdisciplinary teams with shared goals and mutual accountability. A well-run operating room or ambulatory care team depends on the interplay of many roles — surgeons, anesthesiologists, scrub techs, nurses, medical assistants, and care coordinators — each working not only at the top of their license, but also in alignment with professional ethics and mutual trust.

Yet in many systems today, physicians remain buried under tasks that do not require their expertise. EHR inboxes are cluttered with messages that could be triaged by others. Policy changes may restrict support staff from entering orders that clinicians could review and sign. These inefficiencies are not merely workflow flaws; they represent a failure to design for a professional purpose.

To build better care systems, we must do more than redistribute tasks. We must honor the core work of every clinician and ensure that the structures we create support not only efficiency, but also integrity, meaning, and joy in the practice of medicine.

CHAPTER 8

Scope of Practice

"Scope of practice" defines the boundaries of what healthcare professionals are trained and authorized to do. As the complexity of care delivery has increased, the mismatch between what clinicians are trained to do and what they actually spend time doing has grown. This misalignment contributes to inefficiency, clinician burnout, and rising costs.

A medical license grants physicians the legal authority to deliver a broad range of diagnostic, therapeutic, procedural, and palliative services. However, it is every professional's responsibility to only provide services that they are well-trained to do and sufficiently skilled to prevent harm to the patients they care for. Over the last 100 years, this has led to ever-increasing levels of training and sub-specialization as medical knowledge has grown exponentially, Today, specializations center on new technologies (radiology, anesthesiology), age of the patient (pediatrics, geriatrics), organ system (neurology, cardiology, nephrology), disease type (oncology, diabetology), symptom type (pain specialists), and even place where a service is being delivered (SNFists, hospitalists).

Most physicians now undergo a minimum of 11–15 years of education and training, with subspecialists adding additional years beyond that. A single year of internship after graduating from a four-year medical school in the early 20th century has been replaced by an internship and a three- to five-year residency for general specialties such as general surgery, pediatrics, internal medicine, ob-gyn and family medicine, followed by a one- to five-year fellowship for those advancing to subspecialties such as oncology, neurosurgery, and cardiology. Additional training is required for subspecialties such as interventional cardiology, spine surgery, or maternal-fetal medicine.

As the sub-specialization becomes more in-depth, the broad general skills of early medical school training and internships can fade, resulting in an undersupply of physicians and advanced practice providers who can provide basic general medical care.

After completing my internal medicine residency, I became proficient in ICU-level procedures, including lumbar punctures, thoracenteses, central line placements, bone marrow biopsies, and ventilator management. However, as I transitioned into a combined hospital/ambulatory/nursing home practice, those procedural tasks increasingly fell to specialists. Meanwhile, my skills evolved toward outpatient diagnostics, chronic disease management, and minor procedures, demonstrating how the scope of practice adapts to setting and context.

My practice is currently limited to the outpatient ambulatory setting. As a result, my scope of practice has changed. It would be completely inappropriate for me to perform procedures I used to be quite skilled at doing.

The concept of scope of practice is relevant to the problem of differentiating the chores of medicine from the core mission because the chores of providing efficient and effective medical care have changed markedly as sub-specialization has emerged in medical training. Many basic "chores" in medical care fall disproportionately on the shoulders of primary care clinicians, such as signing off on inpatient hospitalists' orders for physical therapy, managing referrals, documenting and managing quality measures for value contracts, and handling medication prior authorizations. On the subspecialty side, prior authorizations for procedures, inpatient admissions, advanced diagnostic testing, and expensive medications are also significantly burdensome.

How many of these chores that are pushed to physicians can be offloaded to other people who have fewer years of training but are familiar with appropriate guidelines and clinical protocols? The scope of practice becomes relevant, as some regulations shift these responsibilities to professionals who might be far more effective using their skills to provide direct medical services.

Part of the politics of this has been complicated by the medical trade organizations' advocacy for limiting the scope of practice of non-physician providers based on their relatively short years of training compared to physicians. This has resulted in several illogical regulatory logjams, such as the requirement that physicians, rather than advanced practice providers, review and sign off on physical therapy orders. During the pandemic, the federal government loosened some of these regulatory barriers, with apparently no adverse effects on patients. In 2025, CMS introduced a new exception to streamline the physical therapy certification process plans of care, further simplifying the certification process.

These administrative burdens — often unrelated to clinical expertise — are forms of scope creep, in which physicians take on tasks that do not require their training. As a more efficient healthcare delivery system is designed around eliminating unnecessary chores from clinical workflows, the scope of practice constraints should be evaluated appropriately. With the advent of near-instantaneous access through artificial intelligence augmented by detailed, evidence-based guidance at the point of care, the scope of practice may evolve to broader roles for generalist physicians and advanced practice providers and fewer subspecialists. If so, the scope of practice and practicing at the top of one's license will rapidly evolve. It may facilitate the efficient delivery of state-of-the-art healthcare services.

To fully realize the potential of scope-of-practice evolution, policymakers must pair technological innovation with regulatory flexibility, ensuring clinicians practice at their highest capacity while shedding unnecessary chores.

CHAPTER 9

Designing the Well-Functioning Clinical Team

A well-functioning healthcare team is built on clearly defined roles and responsibilities. This requires a thoughtful understanding of each team member's training, scope of practice, licensing constraints, and individual skill set. By systematically mapping who does what, how team members interact, and who can serve as backup for whom, organizations can build high-performing clinical teams that optimize both care quality and staff well-being.

Effective workflow design does more than improve efficiency — it also enhances patient safety. Every team member must operate within the boundaries of their competence and training. Well-structured workflows help ensure this, while also reducing burnout, minimizing attrition, and maximizing the contributions of all team members. When tasks are appropriately distributed, clinicians can spend more time practicing at the top of their license and less time burdened by work that others are equally as or better suited to perform.

Team-based care demands adaptability. Many of the traditional hierarchies in medicine — where physicians sit at the top of rigid structures — no longer reflect the reality of how care is delivered. However, this evolution does not require physicians to relinquish leadership. Instead, it calls for physicians to lead differently: by understanding what *must* be done by a physician and what *can* be delegated to other skilled professionals, and by building teams that reflect those insights.

This leadership must operate within the legal framework of state licensing and the enduring cultural norms of medical professionalism: competence, responsibility, integrity, and accountability. The ethical foundation of the physician-patient relationship still rests on the classic virtues of compassion, discernment, trustworthiness, and integrity. These virtues require that harm be avoided — not just through clinical actions, but through the way care teams are structured and led.

Team-based care does not diminish the principles of medical professionalism; when designed well, it reinforces them. By distributing responsibility wisely and respecting each team member's role, modern clinical teams can uphold the profession's deepest values while delivering care that is safer, more efficient, and more humane.

CHAPTER 10

Your Mission Is Your Core

When I asked ChatGPT to generate a sample health system mission statement, it returned a polished, patient-centered message — nearly indistinguishable from many actual statements in use today: "At {Health System Name}, we are dedicated to enhancing the health and well-being of the communities we serve. Our mission is to provide high-quality, accessible, and compassionate healthcare that empowers individuals to lead healthier lives. We strive to innovate and integrate our services, ensuring that every patient receives personalized care based on their unique needs. Through collaboration, education, and a commitment to excellence, we aim to be a trusted partner in health, fostering a healthier future for all."

It is not far from, and occasionally better worded than, the mission statements of various well-known healthcare systems in the United States:

Advocate Health: The mission of Advocate Health Care is to serve the health needs of individuals, families, and communities through a holistic philosophy rooted in our fundamental understanding of human beings as created in the image of God.

Baylor Scott and White: Promotes the well-being of all individuals, families, and communities.

Cleveland Clinic: Caring for life, researching for health, educating those who serve.

Duke Health: Advancing Health Together.

Kaiser Permanente: Kaiser Permanente's mission is to provide high-quality, affordable health care services and improve the health of their members and communities.

Massachusetts General Brigham: Mass General Brigham is committed to serving the community. We are dedicated to enhancing patient care, teaching, and research, and taking a leadership role as an integrated health care system.

Mayo Clinic: Inspiring hope and promoting health through integrated clinical practice, education, and research.

The mission statements of some independent medical groups have a similar tone:

Atlanta Women's Health Group: Our mission is to help empower you, our patients, to take control of your health and well-being.

Austin Regional Clinic: Our mission is to provide coordinated, comprehensive, accessible health care to individuals and families in Central Texas, with sensitivity to the cost of that care. We believe that each doctor/patient relationship is unique.

Holston Medical Group: Holston Medical Group's Mission is to provide quality medical care that exceeds patients' expectations and builds lasting relationships. As a health partner for life, we seek opportunities to build connections and provide support outside the walls of our offices and out in our communities.

Iowa Clinic: To be the healthcare provider of choice for the people of central Iowa by delivering the highest quality of care and service.

Texas Health Care: Texas Health Care's mission and purpose is to create a practice environment that allows our physician member-owners to maximize their time interacting with those who need them the most — their patients — and allows each physician to maintain a sense of professional satisfaction.

Vancouver Clinic: Our mission is to improve the health of our communities by providing high-quality, compassionate care.

Employing over 90,000 physicians and 40,000 advanced practice clinicians, Optum Healthcare is the largest physician employer in the country. Optum is a subsidiary of UnitedHealthcare, the for-profit behemoth that ranks 4th on the Fortune 500 list. The Optum website is quite enthusiastic about its mission:

"We have a bold mission: help people live healthier lives and help make the health system work better for everyone."

Finally, those healthcare organizations that are funded and managed by private equity as an increased share of the market are also focused on worthy missions:

EVP Eyecare: EVP Eyecare's mission is to improve people's lives by providing better vision and outstanding patient experiences.

GI Alliance: GI Alliance's mission is to provide exceptional patient care for gastrointestinal and liver disorders through a patient-first, physician-led approach.

Platinum Dermatology: Platinum Dermatology Partners' mission is to empower the practice of dermatology by creating an exceptional experience for patients, physicians, and all involved in providing the highest level of care.

Each of these provider organizations, whether they are organized as not-for-profit or for-profit, with private investment, public investment, charitable organization, religiously affiliated or not, has a laudable mission focused on high-quality care for patients, and for many, physician and community well-being as well. But if mission alignment were real, why is there so much burnout among front-line clinicians and their staffs?

I am willing to bet that most individuals in these organizations would state that their organization is not adequately fulfilling its mission every day. Approximately half of all physicians in the country report they are burned out, as do 57% of advanced practice clinicians and 60% of nurses. [26,27] While efforts to address this have focused on the individual's well-being, in fact, these rates of burnout are an indictment against the entire health system and will not be resolved until the system itself is fixed.

Burnout is not stress, anxiety, or depression, although it can contribute to these mental health concerns. People who experience burnout often shut down, disconnect. They are not stressed because they no longer care, but because they no longer have the capacity to care.[28]

Burnout is essentially caused by a toxic organizational culture, or, in the case of healthcare, perhaps an entire industry's toxic culture. At the granular level, burnout is caused by a variety of factors, including work overload, lack of control/autonomy, insufficient recognition, a breakdown of the workplace community, a sense of unfairness, and a conflict of values. Studies have shown that burnout often hits hardest in sectors with compassionate employees. People are so committed to the mission that they feel that taking a moment for themselves is selfish or that they are depriving their beneficiaries each minute they don't commit. The World Health Organization recently included burnout in its International Classification of Diseases (ICD-11), stating it "refers specifically to phenomena in the occupational context...a syndrome conceptualized as resulting from chronic workplace stress that has not been successfully managed...." [29] A *Harvard Business*

Review article on burnout notes that those individuals in roles that are "purpose-driven" are at higher risk of burnout.[30]

Much can be done to reconnect healthcare professionals with their passion and energy for their work. Psychologist Abraham Maslow described a hierarchy of human needs that culminates in self-actualization — the realization of one's full potential and purpose. For healthcare professionals, this peak is reached through meaningful clinical relationships, diagnostic mastery, healing, and service — what this book defines as the core of care.

But in today's healthcare environment, clinicians spend much of their time mired in chores: redundant documentation, endless inbox messages, prior authorizations, and administrative bottlenecks. These tasks obstruct the path to self-actualization, draining purpose and driving burnout.

Reconnecting clinicians to their core mission and systematically offloading or redesigning the chores may be the most effective way to restore meaning, joy, and sustainability to clinical work.

CHAPTER 11

What Has To Be Done Where?

Understanding where work must be done — clinically, geographically, and technologically — is fundamental to separating the core mission of healthcare from the chores that obscure it. The physical and institutional structure of healthcare delivery systems has long reflected outdated assumptions about cost, access, and capability. Some work must be done in hospitals and by clinicians, but much can and should be done elsewhere or by others.

HISTORICAL EVOLUTION OF CARE LOCATIONS

The healthcare ecosystem was designed around types of locations where healthcare services are provided. Prior to the 20th century, affluent individuals received healthcare services at home, while those without resources were forced to go to hospitals, which were essentially almshouses for the poor and sick, typically run by religious organizations.

Frequently associated with caring for those wounded in war, hospitals became more secularized and professionalized in the 19th century, particularly after Florence Nightingale pioneered the modern profession of nursing during the Crimean War. She was instrumental in reforming the hospital from primarily being a place where the sick went to die to a place of healing and caring.

By the 20th century, modern hospitals were essential to providing effective healthcare services such as anesthesia and antisepsis. New integrated technologies, such as X-rays and laboratory testing services, require centralized locations in communities for the delivery of state-of-the-art healthcare.

The late Clay Christensen, a Harvard Business School professor most known for his concept of "disruptive innovation," used the "jobs to be done" framework to explain the "why" behind customer behavior. He argued that the hospital's job was to efficiently aggregate healthcare resources in communities at a time when travel was expensive, and technology was becoming less so. He argued that as travel has become much less costly, the need for hospitals as they are currently construed is less obvious.[31]

Certainly, 75 years ago, a large, centralized facility was needed for most laboratory services in a community, but as equipment became cheaper and smaller, much of this need for centralized resources was eliminated, which meant most primary care physicians were able to perform basic lab work with a machine that sits on a tabletop. Similarly, imaging equipment no longer required massive, centralized locations.

THE HOSPITAL BUSINESS MODEL
AND ITS INCENTIVES

As hospitals found their centralized resources competing with businesses that provided similar services in independent physician offices and imaging centers, they lobbied law makers to enact various protective measures, such as certificate of need requirements in order to provide imaging services, Clinical Laboratory Improvement Amendments (CLIA) that set standards for all laboratory testing, and higher reimbursement rates for hospital-based services due to the high cost of providing those services in the hospital location.

Hospital leaders emphasized that their costs of delivery services were higher due to their need to be open 24/7, never turn away a patient in need of emergency care, irrespective of ability to pay, and cross-subsidization of necessary services that are not profitable. This point is valid, but may be less relevant as technology continues to advance, making healthcare less expensive elsewhere.

Currently, healthcare financing greatly advantages the provision of healthcare services in centralized locations. For example, it has typically been far more efficient to monitor many people requiring cardiac monitoring in a single location rather than providing these services in their homes. In fee-for-service medicine, the business model encourages the delivery of as many units of the service one is providing as efficiently as possible, so companies invest in capacity in the form of an increasing number of facilities and an integrated provider network to direct referrals to the business.

THE DISRUPTIVE SHIFT FROM COVID
AND TELEHEALTH

The COVID pandemic required us to quickly rethink how and where healthcare is delivered. The use of telehealth became widespread and necessary when the virus necessitated social distancing in order to slow its spread. This was achieved through video technology that had long been available, and the federal government's lifting of its rule that healthcare be in person in order to get reimbursed.

Overnight, chronic care and urgent care were appropriately provided through televisits, with hospitals being relegated to providing the services that required a facility, such as intensive care and emergency surgery. COVID-19 laid bare how much of healthcare's infrastructure was built on inertia rather than necessity. The crisis didn't just force a new way of working — it revealed how much of our existing system could be reimagined.

What parts of the healthcare system can be redesigned to lower the cost based on facility costs while keeping the necessary services that must be provided in such locations? Administrative tasks do not all have to be provided in centralized healthcare facilities.

EMERGING TECHNOLOGIES AND NEW POSSIBILITIES FOR HOME-BASED CARE

As clinical and administrative healthcare services and work are shifted to lower-cost settings, the healthcare delivery system will need to reevaluate how it covers the still-necessary centralized medical services that hospitals need to provide, including, at least for now, labor and delivery, intensive care, and emergency care.

Much of the hospital's fixed costs are cross-subsidized in complex ways. Disproportionate Share Hospital (DSH) payments are transferred to hospitals that serve a high percentage of Medicaid and uninsured patients. 340B drug programs improve hospital drug costs by mandating drug manufacturers supply drugs at deep discounts, while permitting hospitals to continue to bill at market rates. Facility fees are charged in hospital outpatient departments when physician practices are acquired in addition to professional fees, and commercial insurance rates are often 200-300% higher than Medicare and Medicaid rates to offset losses, but cost-shift to employers.

These mechanisms are intended to preserve essential hospital functions but often distort market incentives, tying the fate of core services to a maze of financial cross-subsidies. As new technologies and business models drive some of the services and much of the costs out of the acute hospital setting, realignment at the policy level to pay the actual costs of necessary services rather than relying on cross-revenue streams could significantly rectify imbalances in healthcare costs all around. Redesigning care delivery also means redesigning how we pay for what matters without hiding core costs behind revenue generated by administrative chores.

The advent of "the internet of things" has given us technology capable of providing sophisticated monitoring services at patients' homes. Services like Dispatch Health send a medical assistant and an advanced practice provider to people's homes with x-ray equipment, basic lab draw equipment, and minor procedure supplies in a van the size of an Amazon delivery vehicle.

Hospital-at-home services now permit patients to receive services previously provided only in the inpatient setting, provided they meet certain criteria for stability. Amazon's Pillpack service is experimenting with drones to deliver prescription medications directly to people's homes, and access to the best specialty care in the world for rare and serious disorders is now available through internet consultation.

These disruptions are built on evolving technologies that permit more convenient, less expensive care in the home rather than in a centralized facility. This begs the question of what all can be done elsewhere and what cannot. For the foreseeable future, we still need centralized locations to treat severe, acute illnesses and trauma, perform surgical procedures, and use other intensive resources in healthcare. But many of the administrative components can be quickly redesigned to lower the costs by separating these core services from the administrative chores that come with them.

By the early 1990s, the concept of outsourcing began to gain traction as hospitals and providers sought to reduce operational costs. Initial efforts focused on administrative tasks, including billing. These outsourced companies, frequently located offshore, offered a skilled workforce at a fraction of the cost compared to the United States. Technological advances, including the rise of the internet, secure data transfer, and electronic health records systems, made it easier for offshore companies to manage billing processes, coding, claims processing, and comprehensive revenue cycle management.

ADMINISTRATIVE CHORES AND THE RISE OF BPO

Business processing outsourcing (BPO) is the practice of contracting specific business processes to third-party service providers. In healthcare, "back office" services like billing are commonly outsourced, but the range of possibilities is much broader. It can include everything from other traditional back-office services like human resources and payroll to "front office services" like customer support.

In healthcare, it may also include prior authorizations, clinical documentation, coding, care coordination, and even clinical services such as virtual clinical support teams. Crucial to all of this is determining what has to be done where. If a task doesn't require a clinician, a hospital, an in-person visit, or even a human being, it should be reassigned. Every layer of complexity that can be safely offloaded, automated, or relocated brings healthcare closer to its mission — and brings clinicians back to the core work that matters most.

CHAPTER 12

Identify the Chores

P olycrisis is a concept used by scholars in systems theory, resilience, and complexity science to frame systemic risk. It describes a situation where multiple global crises interact in complex, compounding ways, leading to far greater challenges than each crisis would pose in isolation, such as the interaction of the global pandemic, climate change, political unrest, and wealth inequality now occurring across the world.[32] The concept emphasizes the interconnectedness and nonlinear effects of these interacting crises and the risk that solving one crisis may worsen another if they are not approached from a systems perspective. The concept can be applied to the healthcare delivery system, which faces its own intersecting crises. But how do we solve our polycrisis?

When you are in the middle of a stressful experience, it is often difficult to imagine an alternative reality. Psychological stress creates physiological responses and emotional pain, but this does not necessarily lead to creative problem-solving. Two of the most familiar metaphors for this phenomenon are characterized in animal stories. The first is the proverbial frog sitting in a pot of water that slowly comes to a boil. The message is that the frog will sit there until it boils to death rather than instinctively jumping out as a frog would do if placed in an already boiling pot of water. The learned helplessness implied in the metaphor is a psychological state that occurs when someone repeatedly faces uncontrollable stressful situations and does not try to change them because they have "learned" that they are helpless, so they no longer try to change the situation (whether true or not).

The second animal metaphor was used by David Foster Wallace in his famous commencement speech at Kenyon College in 2005.[33] Two young fish were swimming along and happened to meet an older fish swimming the other way. The older fish nodded at them and said, "Morning, boys. How's the water?" The two young fish swam on for a bit, then eventually one of them looked at the other and said, "What the hell is water?" Wallace was making the point that somehow the most fundamental aspects of our existence sometimes go unnoticed.

Many of the fundamental aspects of what physicians do when they get up and go to work and see patients all day long are like these two parables: We have learned helplessness and do not understand fundamental aspects of our daily work lives. The polycrisis within the healthcare system engenders this learned helplessness. The key to withdrawing from this state of helplessness is to separate the chores of one's job from its core mission and design solutions for the interconnected dysfunctions produced by the chores. We must parse that which is essential (the core) from that which can be redesigned (chores).

CHORES REQUIRING REINVENTION

Clinical Documentation: Hijacking Time Spent on Patient Care

> **Purpose:** To capture clinically meaningful information, support continuity of care, ensure legal documentation, and enable billing compliance.
>
> **Problem:** Outdated E&M guidelines and rigid formatting have turned documentation into a data-entry burden for physicians—often emphasizing volume over value.
>
> **Solution:** Leverage large language model-based ambient documentation tools, AI-driven clinical decision support, and EHR-integrated automation to shift the physician's role from transcriber to verifier.
>
> **Core vs. Chore Insight:** Documentation is core. Typing, structuring, and redundantly reformatting information? That's chore work.

The purpose of clinical documentation is to convey an accurate representation of a medical service provided in a way that captures meaningful clinical information about the history, objective findings, assessment, and planning, such that clinicians can communicate effectively, thought processes can be recorded, evidence of the clinical encounter can be recorded for billing compliance, and legal requirements can be met.

But fulfilling the purpose does not mean that a physician has to create all the documentation themselves, whether through pen and paper, typing, data entry, dictation, scribing, or AI-generated notes. It does not mean that the 1995/1997 pre-EHR era E&M guidelines that emphasized old clinical documentation formatting, such as 14-point reviews of systems, family, social, and past history, are the proper way to efficiently document in the 2020s, when copy and paste generates such information (and misinformation) without conveying additional value.

The technology available today can allow large language model-built ambient listening technologies to help design notes that perform the essential functions of clinical documentation and, over time, will be able to add clinical decision support built on evidence-based medicine, order entry, and billing and coding, all without the need to turn physicians into data-entry clerks.

Prior Authorization Bureaucracy Masquerading as Clinical Oversight

Purpose: To ensure appropriate use of expensive or potentially unnecessary treatments.

Problem: Current processes create excessive friction, demand manual documentation, and require appeals that waste time and drive burnout.

Solution: Automate prior authorization with AI-based chart abstraction, payer integration, gold-carding for high-performing clinicians, and real-time clinical decision support.

Core vs. Chore Insight: Judging medical necessity is core. Extracting and faxing documentation is not.

The purpose of prior authorization is to prevent physicians from prescribing expensive medications, procedures, or therapies that may not be medically necessary or when alternative, less costly approaches have not been tried first. This purpose is laudable, given the huge amount of non-evidence-based treatments and clinical variations that exist in medical practice. But the current process is deliberately designed to make providing the information about the rationale for a particular therapy as difficult as possible for clinical practices, including demanding prolonged phone calls and requests for excessive amounts of clinical documentation.

A 2024 survey of 1,000 physicians practicing across the United States indicated that prior authorizations impose significant costs on the industry through unnecessary office visits, immediate care visits, and hospitalizations.[34] The survey of 600 specialists and 400 primary care physicians found that on average, physicians' practices complete 39 prior authorizations per physician per week, and physicians and their staff spend 13 hours each week processing prior authorizations. Forty percent of physicians have staff who work exclusively on prior authorizations. Twenty percent of physicians said they always appeal an adverse prior authorization decision; two-thirds said they do not appeal if they do not think the appeal will be successful; more than half said they do not appeal if they have insufficient resources or time. Nine out of 10 reported that the prior authorization process somewhat or significantly increases burnout.

Although the chore of prior authorization can be soul-crushing, it can be redesigned with technology that abstracts the appropriate information from the medical record and transmits it electronically to the payer or proactively prompts physicians to document the appropriate information when prior authorization is likely to be required.

Technology will also make it easier to eliminate the prior authorization requirement for those clinicians who demonstrate cost-effective, evidence-based treatment outcomes through a gold-carding process. Improvements in clinical decision support tools at the point of care can also create easier workflows that provide evidence-based protocols, formulary information, and cost transparency.

Credentialing: Necessary Oversight, Needless Repetition

Purpose: To verify clinician qualifications for licensing, hospital privileges, and insurer networks.

Problem: Manual data entry and duplicative document submission across institutions waste clinician time and introduce administrative drag.

Solution: Use bots and AI to prepopulate credentialing applications, manage renewals, and synchronize data across platforms.

Core vs. Chore Insight: Verification is important. Re-entering the same information across multiple portals? Pure chore.

Credentialing has traditionally required substantial amounts of data entry for clinicians seeking hospital privileges, payment from insurers, and medical licensing. New technology built with large language models and bots can now upload the redundant information required for all of these efforts, create appropriate forms in real time, and populate the data, saving countless hours and administrative burden. By redesigning this chore, we can return clinicians to their core mission.

Coding: Complexity Without Clinical Value

Purpose: To document and categorize services for reimbursement and population health risk adjustment.

Problem: Requires clinicians to memorize nuanced coding rules, which diverts focus from work.

Solution: Automated coding engines embedded in EHRs, supported by real-time prompts and LLM-based validation of HCC documentation.

Core vs. Chore Insight: Capturing the essence of care is core. Navigating CPT/HCC minutiae? Chore.

Physicians have been burdened with the ever-increasingly complex chore of coding for billing purposes, such that an entire industry now exists that will review medical records to confirm medical documentation meets billing criteria from a compliance and revenue perspective. Technology is being developed that will identify whether clinical documentation meets the required elements for evaluation and management and procedure coding autonomously.

Likewise, the hierarchical condition category (HCC) coding that is important in identifying who the sickest patients are for population health and value-based care contracts can be redesigned with technology that determines whether these conditions are appropriately flagged within the context of the MEAT criteria (monitored, evaluated, assessed, and treated rather than just coded).

Inbox Management: A Digital Dumping Ground

Purpose: To manage patient inquiries, prescription refills, results, and care coordination.

Problem: Physicians are flooded with redundant messages, system-generated alerts, and non-clinical tasks, much of which could be triaged.

Solution: Protocol-driven triage teams, AI-generated auto-responses, role-based routing, and ambient assistants that reduce unnecessary notifications.

Core vs. Chore Insight: Responding to urgent clinical questions is a core task. Deleting duplicate refill confirmations isn't.

In the past, my clinical workflows with respect to evaluating information were people-dependent and protected my clinical time. Patients who called in via a telephone spoke to someone at the front desk who determined whether the issue was something they could address, like making an appointment, or triaged it to the registered nurse who called the patient to provide information about test results and studies, ready prescription refills for my approval, communicate with a local pharmacist, and complete the necessary paperwork for prior authorizations, physical therapy orders, etc. for me to sign.

Then came electronic health records. Many of these tasks were made electronic and designed for a quick push of a button to go directly to me. As large health systems bought previously private practices, almost all of the work that was previously done by the clinical staff was deemed to be beyond the "scope" of the medical assistants. Workflows evolved that pushed more and more of this directly to clinicians, with burnout rising across medical specialties accordingly.

When COVID hit, patients could communicate directly with physicians through the portals — a practice driven by telehealth and the need for remote access to health information. In 2020, approximately 38% of patients accessed their medical practices through patient portals. By 2022, this had increased to 57%.[35] Many patients began using the portal for casual conversations with their physicians, greatly increasing the burden of delivering care. The type of tasks in the inbox that previously would have been handled by the staff became new work for clinicians themselves.

In 2020, the Centers for Medicare and Medicaid Services introduced billing codes that allow providers to be reimbursed for digital evaluations. As a result, many prominent health systems have adopted the practice of billing for these services, including the Cleveland Clinic, Johns Hopkins Medicine, University of Washington Medicine, Novant Health, Houston Methodist, MultiCare, and Northwestern Medicine.

The inbox for most physicians has become an undifferentiated nightmare of endless tasks and communication requirements that demand substantial time and create significant new and excessive work. However, inbox solutions can be built that allow others to do much of this work. These solutions are built upon protocols that do not burden the physicians with the keypunch work of order entry and chatty back-and-forths with patients about medical questions that do not require physician expertise.

IKS Health found that up to 40% of inbox messaging from patients to clinics was inquiries about whether they had received messages about prescription refills from the pharmacy or had read a previous message. Simply sending an electronic message back acknowledging receipt of such messages can eliminate a substantial inbox burden, as can automated messaging about normal lab results, referrals, appointments, and prescription refills.

Prescription Refills: Automate the Routine

Purpose: To ensure safe, accurate continuation of necessary medications.

Problem: Physicians must often manually verify history, labs, and insurance details — steps that can be standardized.

Solution: Refill workflows can be governed by protocols, managed by care teams, or queued for physician review only when necessary.

Core vs. Chore Insight: Reviewing complex cases for med reconciliation is core. Approving standard chronic meds repeatedly is chore work.

The workflows associated with incoming messages for prescription refills can be developed such that any necessary diagnostic testing, office visit requirements, drug-drug interactions, and formulary changes can be developed by protocol without physicians having to look up the information, and the prescriptions can be refilled directly by protocol or teed up in the electronic health record for the physician for final sign-off. If properly designed, with the right technology and trained personnel, much of this work can be done outside the confines of the clinical office.

Patient Communication: Respect the Core, Redesign the Channel

Purpose: To support continuity, education, and trust in the doctor-patient relationship.

Problem: Unfiltered portal messages and expectations for immediate replies are overwhelming physicians, especially in primary care.

Solution: Use message filtering, support teams, tiered response protocols, and AI-generated responses for routine inquiries.

Core vs. Chore Insight: Connecting with patients in meaningful ways is core. Managing all communication volume personally is an unsustainable chore.

In the past, physicians were mostly shielded from routine communication with patients by layers of office staff who triaged communication based upon medical urgency. However, patients are accustomed to instant communication with other service providers 24/7 in real time and expect ongoing and immediate communication back with their clinicians. Much of this communication falls on the shoulders of the primary care staff. Specialists seem to have fewer inbox communication requests from patients and fewer expectations of instant communication back. With a global human work force and automated technologies and workflows, much of this type of work can be handled by teams and technology rather than the inappropriate focus on the primary care physician as the endpoint of all clinical workflow.

CHAPTER 13

Pajama Time Is Evil

The term "pajama time" offends me. Pajama time is a misleading euphemism for unpaid clerical labor imposed on physicians after hours. Far from cozy productivity in fuzzy slippers, this is a prime example of how core clinical work is buried under the burden of chore — data entry, inbox triage, and bureaucratic mandates that sap meaning from the practice of medicine. This term refers to work performed after hours and at home by physicians in their electronic health records.

But the image of physicians sitting at home in front of their laptops, perhaps wearing their comfy pajamas and fuzzy slippers, is disarmingly inappropriate. "Work after work," a more accurate description, is a major contributor to physician burnout, stealing personal and family time. Physicians who reported marginal time for clinical documentation had 2.8 times the odds of burnout compared to those reporting sufficient time. Physicians who reported moderately high/excess time on EHRs at home had 1.9 times the odds of burnout compared to those with minimal/no EHR use at home.[36]

Of the 1,792 Rhode Island physicians surveyed in the study, 70% reported health information technology-related stress, with those with time pressures for documentation or those doing excessive "work after hours" on their EHR at home having twice the odds of burnout compared to physicians who did not face these challenges.

Primary care physicians spend nearly two hours on EHR tasks for each hour of direct patient care during and after clinic hours. These tasks include clerical and administrative jobs such as documentation, order entry, billing and coding, and system security, accounting for half the total EHR time, with inbox management accounting for another 24%.[37] Physicians in ambulatory settings spend more time working in the electronic health record after hours and on unscheduled days, including weekends, than physicians who work in inpatient settings, with physicians with more clinical time disproportionately burdened by work after work. Physicians who spend more than four scheduled days per week in the clinic spend an average of 2.8 hours on the EHR per unscheduled day.

Christine Sinsky, MD, a co-author of the study, points out that increasing requirements and regulations have fundamentally changed the nature of a physician's work, with "work previously done by other team members having been shifted to the physician in the EHR."[38]

The fact that both Epic and Cerner — the dominant EHR vendors — have built-in tools to measure after-hours work (with names like 'Pajama Time' and 'Work Outside of Scheduled Hours') underscores how deeply this chore has been institutionalized. Epic uses its Signal tool to measure "Time Outside Scheduled Hours (TOSH)," "Time on Unscheduled Days (TUSD)," and "Pajama Time" to capture time on weekends and weekdays outside 7:00 am to 5:30 pm. Cerner's EHR tracks after-hours workload, including time spent on documentation, reviewing charts, and responding to messages with a tool called "Lights On Network" that has a metric called "Work Outside of Scheduled Hours," or WOSH. The very fact that these two dominant EHRs have tools to track these metrics implies these vendors acknowledge these after-work requirements.[39]

Across all ambulatory specialties, a significant amount of that time is spent outside of scheduled clinical hours, according to a survey of 200,000 physicians in 2021, using Epic System's Signal platform. This study showed that primary care physicians are spending an average of 2.7 hours PER DAY of their personal time on the electronic health record outside of patient appointments.

Specialties with the greatest amount of time working in the EHRs per eight hours of scheduled patient time were:

• Infectious diseases: 8.4 hours
• Endocrinology: 7.7 hours
• Nephrology: 7.5 hours
• Primary Care: 7.3 hours
• Hematology: 7.2 hours

These specialties care for patients with a high level of complexity with multiple medical conditions requiring more documentation, more orders, and more communication between the patient and care team between visits, so the inbox time is also the highest among these five specialties.[40]

Surgical specialists spend an average of 16 minutes per day after hours on documenting notes, clinical review, order entry, and responding to team and system messages, compared to medical specialists (24.8 minutes) and primary care physicians 51.5 minutes . Primary care clinicians received more than twice as many team-derived messages, five times as many patient messages, and 15 times as many prescription messages each day compared to surgical colleagues.[41] However, higher levels of EHR stress are associated with higher levels of burnout among physicians in *all* specialties; higher levels of prescription authorization are associated with higher odds of burnout.[42]

These statistics represent more than lost time — they represent missed soccer games, hurried dinners, little rest, and physician exhaustion that spills over into patient care the next day. Physicians have always worked long hours to care for patients, but in the past, these hours were primarily focused on direct patient care through on-call access, emergency department coverage, and home and skilled nursing facility visits.

With the reorganization of medical care into narrower location-specific specialties and the introduction of after-hours triage services, this work has diminished, but it has been replaced by the dissatisfactory work of clerical data entry and clinical documentation. With that substitution came increased levels of physician burnout and a decreased interest in general internal medicine, family medicine, and pediatrics among medical students, such that we now have a shortage of primary care access for patients.

Physicians in primary care are paid less, experience more burnout, work longer hours, and have substantially more pajama time. Primary care is not just undervalued — it is under siege. The relentless burden of after-hours administrative work is systematically discouraging young physicians from entering these essential fields. It is the exploitation of a critical professional workforce that may be a primary reason health outcomes in the United States are substandard compared to the rest of the developed world. Primary care is the only healthcare component in which an increased supply is associated with better population health and more equitable outcomes.[43]

In the United States, 84 million people live in areas where there is a shortage of primary care professionals.[44] For more than 10 years, primary care residency programs have not kept up with primary care workforce needs.[45] This shortage is accelerating due to retirement, burnout, and a reduction of clinical hours.[46] Although "pajama time" is not measured directly in these analyses, burnout is, and the inappropriate exploitation of physicians' personal time is no doubt contributing to the primary care shortage. Additionally, the "chores" associated with clinical documentation and order entry — inbox management — reduce in-clinic time by substituting direct patient interaction with administrative tasks. Research shows that for patients, improved primary care translates into 33% lower healthcare costs and 19% lower odds of dying prematurely compared to those who see only a specialist.[47] Eliminating pajama time could strengthen primary care considerably and reduce the expected shortage of 22,000–35,000 primary care physicians by 2033.

CHAPTER 14

Platforms Can Diminish Chores

B uzzwords in healthcare often reflect shifts in policy, payment, or technology. In the 1980s, physicians were typically referred to by specialty — internist, pediatrician, family doctor. But as managed care took hold in the 1990s, the term "primary care physician" (PCP) emerged, driven by the need to control specialist utilization through tiered copays.

Around that same time, the buzzwords "clinically integrated networks" (CINs) and "integrated physician organizations" (IPOs) defined early attempts at physician-hospital alignment. These kinds of changes in terms are almost always related to a change in the payment system rather than a change in medical discipline or learning.

Managed care created a system to control utilization of expensive specialist services by differentiating the co-pay amounts that patients were responsible for paying by categories of PCP/specialty. In the 1990s, hospitals and independent affiliated physicians were trying to figure out how to work together while maintaining their current business models, and the concept of "clinically integrated networks" was devised, which allowed a loose affiliation of physicians to organize with their local hospitals for bargaining purposes.

A few healthcare consultants got wealthy going all over the country advising PCPs to organize into one IPO, specialists into another IPO, and then form their CIN with the hospital in a "joint venture."

Other buzzwords through the years have included "value-based care," "social determinants of health," "integrative healthcare," "complementary medicine," "meaningful use," "precision medicine," "whole-person care," "patient engagement," "evidence-based medicine," "population health," "comprehensive care," "activities of daily living," "patient centered care," "medical home," and "comprehensive medication management."

Lately, the healthcare buzzwords are less directed at business models and healthcare models and more at digital technology and how it has impacted healthcare. Terms include "point solution," "full-stack solution," "asynchronous care," "digital front door," "big data," "telemedicine," "digital transformation," "artificial intelligence," "interoperability," and "consumerism," although "payvider" is also now in the vernacular.

All of these buzzwords emerged as a result of a change in technology and the healthcare business model. Among physicians, this occurred, too. Internal medicine, which is my specialty, is a discipline in medicine that is focused on the diagnosis and treatment of medical conditions in adult patients, focusing on their "internal" organ systems in a comprehensive way. The subdivision of the discipline into medical specialties occurred as medical science expanded, and certain physicians focused their practices entirely on a single organ system. In contrast, many of the new ways that internal medicine has been renamed with buzzwords are not about medical training, but rather a location in which one practices internal medicine (hospitalist, SNFist) or a particular model of care (extensivists).

One of today's dominant healthcare buzzwords that originated in the tech field and is now a part of healthcare terminology is "platform." A platform is a business model that facilitates interactions between participants (patients, clinicians, payers) in ways that reduce friction and enable scaled value exchange.

John Hagel describes four types of platforms:[48]

1. **Aggregation**. The purpose is to bring together a wide array of resources or participants for transactions. Examples: online appointment schedulers, provider directories, and marketplaces for services.
2. **Social**. The purpose is to connect individuals with shared interests. Examples: peer-to-peer support communities and clinician networks.
3. **Mobilization**. The purpose is to enable coordinated action to achieve shared goals. Examples: supply chain networks and clinical research collaborations.
4. **Learning**. The purpose is to facilitate rapid knowledge-sharing and improvement over time. Examples: AI-driven clinical decision support, shared quality dashboards, and learning health systems.

Platforms differ from traditional tools in that they enable relationships and exchanges, not just transactions. As healthcare evolves, moving from siloed systems to true platforms can reduce administrative "chores" and restore focus to the clinical "core."

Bain and Company have pointed out that seven of the 10 largest companies in the world are powered by platforms: Microsoft, Apple, Alphabet, Amazon, Meta, NVIDIA, and Tencent.[49] The same has not been true for healthcare, where point solutions and manual transactions connect disparate entities in the industry. Platforms have been harder to build and scale in healthcare due to its fragmented, complex, and highly regulated nature. The pricing models are opaque, and the economic incentives are misaligned. However, the move to value-based care, consumerism, the federal mandate for interoperability, and the expansion of virtual and home-based care models are starting to break down the barriers to developing functional, efficient healthcare platform models.[50]

The federally mandated Fast Healthcare Interoperability Resources (FHIR) standard for data exchange allows vendors to share information, enabling healthcare systems to get a more complete view of their patients and business processes. The platform business model allows a central framework to orchestrate the exchange of value among external parties, acting as a conduit that connects buyers and sellers of goods and services, without requiring businesses to directly own these commodities.[51]

Unlike the legacy systems designed around transactional billing and siloed documentation — what I call "chore-generating workflows" — platforms are designed to orchestrate relationships, automate non-core tasks, and allow clinicians to focus on their true mission: care delivery. They are not just digital solutions, but systemic redesigns that shift how work gets done.

For the platform business model to reshape the healthcare landscape, one must deeply understand the current healthcare industry workflows. Many of these workflows have been designed for the transactions necessary in a non-connected transactional environment and make up a large portion of the "chores" that increasingly burden medical practices, such that they cannot focus efficiently on their core mission. The dysfunctional designs of many healthcare information systems are the result of these chores being transactional in nature and lacking interoperability.

Every new healthcare technology becomes superimposed on the old transactional workflows and business models, often as "point solutions" used as workarounds, such that transactional business processes are engendered. Most electronic health records are essentially glorified billing systems, built to serve the fee-for-service model, not to reduce clinician toil. A true healthcare platform, by contrast, enables seamless data exchange, intelligent automation, and collaborative workflows that remove unnecessary steps rather than digitize them.

The development of functional platforms built on fee-for-service payment models are set up to solve many of the burnout, access, cost, and quality challenges the industry continues to face. For healthcare to truly evolve, we must stop layering new digital point solutions on top of broken processes. We need platform-based redesigns that shift the locus of work, eliminate redundant chores, and free clinicians to practice at the top of their license. Only then can we escape the cycle of burnout and deliver the care our missions promise.

CHAPTER 15

The Purpose of Clinical Documentation and Its Devolution

When Lawrence Weed introduced the problem-oriented medical record (POMR) in a landmark 1968 *New England Journal of Medicine* article, he emphasized that the initial collection of clinical data should be "as significant and complete as possible," provided it did not create undue discomfort, danger, or cost to the patient. He also championed the use of technology to streamline this process, writing that "useful historical data can be acquired and stored cheaply, completely and accurately by new computer and interviewing techniques WITHOUT THE USE OF EXPENSIVE PHYSICIAN TIME [emphasis mine]."[52] Nearly six decades later, that last clause — "without the use of expensive physician time" — has been all but forgotten.

Instead of relieving clinicians of redundant tasks, documentation has become a bloated, burdensome chore that siphons time and energy away from meaningful clinical work. At its core, the purpose of clinical documentation is to comprehensively record a patient's medical history, diagnoses, treatments, and outcomes, ensuring continuity of care, facilitating informed decision-making, and supporting communication across the care team. However, this foundational purpose has been diluted by secondary imperatives, namely, billing optimization and legal risk mitigation. Over time, the clinical record has evolved from a tool for patient care to a defensive artifact and billing ledger.

In theory, clinical documentation should serve to illuminate the clinical narrative, connecting symptoms, assessments, and plans in a coherent arc across time and touchpoints. In practice, it has become a compliance exercise. To maximize reimbursement, clinicians are required to produce elaborate documentation that supports billing codes, often prioritizing volume of information over clinical relevance. Simultaneously, fear of litigation fuels a culture of defensive charting, contributing to "note bloat" and cognitive overload for both the writer and the reader.

The advent of value-based care added another layer of complexity. To capture quality metrics and ensure appropriate risk adjustment, clinicians are now responsible for documenting granular clinical processes and coding comorbidities to reflect medical complexity. Unfortunately, these requirements are often grafted onto already busy visits, transforming documentation into a proxy for performance rather than a tool for patient-centered care. Longitudinal care planning — essential to managing chronic illness — has become especially hard to operationalize within episodic encounters.

By 2015, the burden of documentation had reached such extremes that the American College of Physicians issued a position paper calling for urgent reform. The ACP reminded the profession that documentation was originally intended to support care coordination and clinical reasoning — not to serve external stakeholders. Yet, the rise of electronic health records introduced new dysfunctions: note bloat, irrelevant template-generated content, and excessive copying and pasting.

The 1995 and 1997 Evaluation and Management (E/M) coding guidelines — intended to quantify cognitive services — further distorted the purpose of documentation. Instead of validating what physicians *did*, they prioritized what physicians *wrote*, leading to a compliance-first mindset. As the ACP warned, this has created "an imbalance of values, with coding and compliance trumping clarity and conciseness," fostering a "gotcha" culture that erodes professionalism and saps meaning from the practice of medicine.[53]

Clinical documentation, once a core tool of medical reasoning and care coordination, has been hijacked by external incentives and turned into a chore. Its original function — to serve the patient and support the care team — must be restored. Leveraging modern technologies like AI-assisted ambient documentation and clinical decision support can help reclaim physician time and refocus clinical attention on what matters most: the patient.

CHAPTER 16

Clinical Documentation Is a Chore

Once a tool for recording meaningful patient encounters, clinical documentation has evolved into a sprawling set of administrative chores that extend far beyond the core task of capturing clinical care. Today's electronic health records impose layers of administrative burden — from billing optimization and legal defensiveness to quality tracking and data mining — that obscure the original clinical purpose of documentation.

The electronic health record now includes such functions and tasks as registries, portals, connected home monitoring devices, patient and provider-controlled mobile devices, and inbox management functions. The medical record has also become a legal document with requirements for non-modification and retention, and "the defined work product for which physicians are paid."[53]

The ease of the copy and paste function allows the carry forward of extensive documentation, providing no additional relevant information other than meeting higher reimbursement requirements for revenue generation purposes, and encourages outright fraud of what was actually performed as part of the clinical interaction.

Backfilling default boilerplate negative findings is time-consuming with handwritten medical records, but easy and fast with electronic health records. Electronic health records can support a higher billing code level without the accusation or appearance of fraud, just by providing an easier method for clinical coding support. Electronic health records also drive the focus on structured data, which requires significant data entry requirements of clinicians for purposes of automating clinical decision support and extracting data for quality measures in pay-for-performance contracts.

The Centers for Medicare & Medicaid Services (CMS) warns that "cloned" documentation — verbatim repetition of prior notes — may indicate fraud or misuse, emphasizing that billing must reflect actual, distinct medical necessity. Yet EHR design makes cloning both tempting and nearly unavoidable. CMS has emphasized that "documentation is considered cloned when each entry in the medical record for a beneficiary is worded exactly like or similar to the previous entries. Cloning of documentation is considered a misrepresentation of the medical necessity requirement for covered services."[54]

Contemporary clinical documentation complexity is driven by new requirements not previously performed by physicians, including completion of medication reconciliation, reviewing often voluminous amounts of outside data, maintaining accurate, updated clinical problem lists, documentation for prior authorization purposes, tracking quality initiatives, tracking public health initiatives, and specific documentation for clinical research. Because current EHRs lack role-based flexibility, physicians end up performing tasks that could — and should — be done by others, turning highly trained clinicians into glorified data entry clerks.

These mounting burdens are compounded by a pervasive culture of documentation shaming. The first time I heard a medical coder say "if it wasn't documented it wasn't done" I was not nearly as offended as the 50th time I heard it, usually from someone in the front of a room with a PowerPoint deck wagging a scolding finger to a room of physicians, focused on frightening them about their risk of medical malpractice with poor clinical documentation, compliance and coding fraud, or "leaving money on the table."

Unfortunately, clinical documentation has led to epidemic burnout, especially among primary care physicians; the medical documentation itself is much worse. My early years in practice were paper-based, but efficient. A simple orange cover sheet recorded the essentials, including active problems, immunizations, allergies, medications, and demographic information, followed by tab sections with medical notes, labs, imaging, consultation notes, and hospital discharge summaries in chronological order. Clinical notes were legible, focused, and easy to navigate.

Today, even finding the relevant information can feel like wading through a bureaucratic swamp. But some things have definitely improved with the integrated electronic health information. The lack of access to my medical partners' patients' clinical records was always difficult when I was on call for a long weekend. Occasionally, I would come into the office to review these records before going to the hospital to see the inpatient records when I was called to the hospital to admit one of their patients.

With the advent of electronic medical records, I was able to see the work of my specialist colleagues instantaneously, which helped with care coordination and prevented unnecessary testing. I no longer had to see a patient in the hospital in the middle of the night with minimal background information. But that has evolved into an absolute nightmare.

When I see a patient in the office now, there are flashing warnings of various "care gaps," many of which are inaccurate, and I cannot confirm without searching through the chart. A drop-down in front of the patient's chart demands I either document HCC codes that have not been documented yet this year in order to receive higher reimbursement from risk-adjusted payments from Medicare or justify why I am not doing so.

Data indicate that more than half of a primary care physician's clinic time is focused on interacting with the requirements of the electronic health record rather than providing actual patient care. Clinical documentation has devolved into a bloated, performative exercise — more about regulatory compliance and billing optimization than patient care. What used to take me a few seconds to document now requires minutes, as my institution also demands that all orders be entered by the clinician rather than through orders given verbally or in writing to medical assistants. When physicians are reduced to keystroke technicians, the core of medicine — clinical judgment, human connection, healing — is displaced by administrative noise.

CHAPTER 17

Don't Let Clinical Decision Support Become a Chore

The health system where I see patients one weekend a month is a behemoth. It is the fifth-largest nonprofit integrated health system in the nation, with annual revenue exceeding $27 billion, 1,000 sites of care, 67 hospitals, 21,000 physicians, and 42,000 nurses. It spans six states in the Southeast and Midwest and includes a world-class academic medical center. Its resources are massive.

We practice medicine using Epic, another behemoth, with annual revenues of around $5 billion. Epic stores the medical records of 78% of U.S. patients and over 3% of the global population. It holds 60% of the market share among U.S. health systems and academic medical centers, covering 39% of the acute care hospital market and over 305 million patients.[55] Companies of this size have the capacity to dramatically improve the cost, quality, efficiency, and experience of care — if leadership aligns those goals with system design.

There has been criticism, however, that health systems and EHR vendors too often prioritize market share and revenue optimization. Robert Kuttner, writing in *The American Prospect*, argues Epic's dominance is partly due to its ability to facilitate upcoding.[56] Between 2014 and 2019, the U.S. Department of Health and Human Services found that inpatient stays billed at the highest severity level increased by nearly 20%. Many argue this financial orientation fuels documentation bloat and unnecessary data entry — especially by physicians. Clinicians are now spending roughly two hours documenting for every one hour of direct patient care, much of it after hours, and much of it irrelevant to actual clinical care.

After a recent EHR system upgrade in my clinic, I encountered new clinical decision support reminders. One flagged a patient as having chronic obstructive pulmonary disease (COPD) and nudged me to order a spirometry test, stating that failure to do so annually constituted "poor quality." But the patient didn't have COPD. I had to comb through the chart to verify this, losing valuable time. It's likely the system had picked up an incorrect data point and triggered the reminder based on an imprecise algorithm — an attempt at evidence-based decision support that missed the evidence and failed to support the decision. Worse, it added to my cognitive load with no clinical value.

Accurate clinical decision support is essential. But it must be based on validated criteria and implemented through intelligent workflows. A more effective population health-based approach to the problem is to identify in the clinical chart signs/symptoms/risk factors for COPD and have a CAP-TURE questionnaire administered to the patient, not necessarily at the point of care.[56] For those patients who then appear to meet the need to have the diagnosis of COPD established, an office visit with an internist or family physician could be made proactively.

Automatically generated clinical note templates in the EHR could utilize clinical decision support tools that ensure the other appropriate tests beyond a basic spirometry were also ordered as part of evidence-based medicine guidelines, such as a CBC to assess for anemia, assessment of electrolytes and kidney function, thyroid function testing, a plasma BNP to rule out congestive heart failure, a chest x-ray to evaluate for alternative parenchymal lung disease. Then the current guideline-based treatments could be embedded into standard order sets, and the annual spirometry reevaluation exam could be automated and based on the patient needing to be seen by a physician.

This supports evidence-based care without burdening the physician with detective work in a 20-minute visit.

Unfortunately, that's not how many EHRs are designed. There's a reluctance to automate population-based care workflows, often due to concerns about "practicing medicine" through algorithms, liability fears, and misaligned incentives under RVU-based payment models. Instead, vague alerts and nudge reminders are pushed to individual physicians, creating more work, not less.

Another example: I recently received a pop-up suggesting referral of a patient for Lynch syndrome genetic counseling. The chart gave no clear reason. Lynch syndrome is rare, affecting about 0.36% of the population, and should only be considered under specific criteria (Amsterdam II).[58] Seven of my patients triggered the alert during the two weeks the alert was activated. None of them met the criteria. I had to manually confirm this by reviewing family history in the chart and with the patient. This misfire not only wasted my time, but it also risked overloading a scarce clinical resource: genetic counselors. A more effective clinical decision support alert would explain, *"This patient meets Amsterdam II criteria based on [specific data]. Consider genetic testing for MLH1, MSH2, MSH6, PMS2, or EPCAM. Referral to a genetic counselor may support shared decision-making."*

The core issue is not that clinical decision support is bad — it's that poorly designed support becomes another chore. The explosion of clinical knowledge and growing expectations for "gap closure" through pop-ups and alerts have made it impossible for physicians to manage without intelligent automation and team-based workflows. The solution is not to ignore best practices but to integrate them into systems that reduce friction and focus physician time on high-value clinical work.

We must build clinical decision support tools that:

- Are grounded in evidence-based guidelines.
- Offer specificity, not vague nudges.
- Support exception management instead of requiring manual review of every case.
- Operate across population health workflows, not just at the point of care.
- Can be managed longitudinally by care teams and not solely by physicians.

Only then can we remove this particular chore and return clinical decision support to its rightful role as a core enabler of better care.

The chores of primary care that result from the even-increasing amount of medical knowledge on what constitutes best care that cannot possibly be accommodated with thousands of care gap messages and patients safety popups could be greatly reduced by properly designed clinical decision support that is built on evidence-based guidelines, deeply clinical criteria (Amsterdam criteria not family history of colon cancer) and population based work flows that populated clinical documentation templates designed to capture best practices and clinical chores that don't have to be performed by the clinicians at the point-of-care elsewhere, through automated tools, and clinical coworkers who have longitudinal workflows and care plans not built around the tyranny of the clinical visit. When thoughtfully designed and supported by appropriate workflows and team roles, clinical decision support can remove chore-like tasks from physicians and allow them to focus on complex decision-making that truly requires their expertise.

CHAPTER 18

When Did Primary Care Become Just Screening and Referring?

Primary care used to mean continuity, comprehensiveness, relationships, and trust. Today, it too often resembles administrative triage — a fragmented, click-driven exercise in documentation and referral.

Once upon a time, my medical practice primarily involved diagnosing and treating adult patients with acute and chronic medical conditions in inpatient, outpatient, and nursing home settings. I could see 25 patients a day, on average, took night calls, raised my family, ran a medical group, and got plenty of sleep, exercise, and reading time. There were times when I was very tired from it all, and certainly, my family will tell you that at times, I was particularly cranky, but I was never in any way close to being what is now called "burned out." I was not special. Medicine, as practiced 30 years ago, was different from what it is now. Somewhere along the way, the nature of work expected of a general internist changed.

The electronic health record is designed mostly for me to click a thousand clicks and prescribe pills, order tests, and as quickly as possible refer to a specialist. I no longer perform lumbar punctures, thoracentesis, bone marrow biopsies, exercise stress tests, and flexible sigmoidoscopies, place central lines, admit patients to the hospital, make house calls, or see patients in the emergency department.

The large health system I work for has removed the office spirometry from the clinical practice site, so that it must now be done not at the point of care, but by way of a referral to the pulmonary practice. Even simple tools like a microscope are now restricted, requiring me to pass a quarterly test just to maintain CLIA-waived lab status. I still inject joints for my patients when needed, provided I can find the supplies to do so, and will do small skin biopsies and cryotherapy, and perform pap smears when supplies are available for me to do so.

What used to be routine aspects of primary care are now nearly impossible — not because they're obsolete, but because the system has been redesigned to obstruct them. The system has been redesigned for me to focus on screening, hunting down HCC codes for higher billing for the system, and entering as much data as possible into the system, barely giving me adequate time to really take care of my patients.

I work in the clinic one weekend a month, so the system is not set up to accommodate my idiosyncratic urge to practice comprehensive internal medicine, and most of the other providers in the space there during the weekdays do none of the procedures I am comfortable doing and refer them out to specialty practices.

I am not the only primary care physician who feels this way. Landon and colleagues recently described the current plight of primary care as "a death by a thousand cuts, a crushing weight of nonclinical demands." They stress that "PCPs have found themselves spending more and more time functioning as de facto administrative assistants," such that their central role in providing comprehensive care is at risk from the escalating volume of administrative tasks that are unsustainable. These tasks range from billing documentation requirements to responding to airlines requiring confirmation that someone needs an emotional support dog to direct patient requests on portals to being the one primarily responsible for "mind-numbing amounts of data entry" to being the "administrator-in-chief" of organizing most aspects of the patient's medical record.[59]

What used to be routine parts of primary care are now nearly impossible — not because they're obsolete, but because the system has been redesigned to obstruct them. When did the work of primary care become about data entry, screening, and referring, and not about practicing good internal medicine? It has been a slow, gradual process built on poorly designed technology and a poorly designed payment system that is in desperate need of reform. Redesign will require many changes.

The first change is to take the nonsensical chores off the backs of physicians and give them the finances, time, and infrastructure to resume the practice of real medicine. If we want to save primary care, we give physicians the time, tools, and trust to do what they were trained to do: heal.

CHAPTER 19

Reclaiming the Core

The stories and data in this section paint a clear picture: Physicians are being buried under a mountain of tasks that have little to do with why they went into medicine. What was once a profession centered on relationships, critical thinking, and hands-on care has been restructured into a fragmented, bureaucratic system that prioritizes data entry and compliance over discernment and healing.

The cumulative weight of the chores — documentation, inbox management, prior authorizations, referrals, coding, screening checklists — has transformed how clinicians spend their time, how they connect with patients, and how they experience their own sense of purpose. We now find ourselves in a healthcare system that tolerates burnout as collateral damage, treats clinical time as a billing opportunity, and fails to invest in what matters most: the relationship between the patient and a physician equipped to care.

But it doesn't have to be this way. If we are willing to separate the core from the chore, if we design our workflows around human beings rather than billing systems, and if we align our technologies and teams around what actually creates value in care, we can reclaim the meaning, joy, and sustainability of practicing medicine.

In Part Two, we'll explore how to do just that: apply human-centered design, team-based care models, and new workflows to rebuild healthcare around its core mission of caring for people.

Human-Centered Design Will Improve Healthcare

Rebuilding Healthcare

"Human centeredness asserts firstly that we must always put people before machines, however complex or elegant that machine might be, and, secondly, it marvels and delights at the ability and ingenuity of human beings. The Human Centered systems movement looks sensitively at these forms of science and technology which meet our cultural, historical, and societal requirements, and seeks to develop more appropriate forms of technology to meet our long-term aspirations. In the Human Centered System, there exists a symbiotic relation between the human and the machine, in which the human being would handle the qualitative subjective judgements and the machine the quantitative elements. It involves a radical redesign of the interface technologies and at a philosophical level, the objective is to provide tools (in the Heidegger sense) which would support human skill and ingenuity rather than machines which would object to that knowledge."[60]

The International Organization for Standardization (ISO) standard 9241-210:2019 defines human-centered design as:

1. An explicit understanding of users, tasks, and environments, the context of use.
2. The involvement of users throughout design and development.
3. A design driven and refined by human-centered evaluation.
4. An interactive process whereby a prototype is designed, tested, and modified, addressing the whole user experience.
5. A design team that includes multidisciplinary skills and perspectives.

Human-centered design is an approach to problem-solving that emphasizes the human perspective in all steps of the design process, in order to make systems, products, and technologies as usable and useful as possible. The International Organization for Standardization (ISO) has adopted human-centered design as one of its standards that covers almost all aspects of technology and manufacturing:

"Human-centered design is an approach to interactive systems development that aims to make systems usable and useful by focusing on the users, their needs and requirements, and by applying human/factors/ergonomics, and usability knowledge and techniques. This approach enhances effectiveness and efficiency, improves human well-being, user satisfaction, accessibility, and sustainability; and counteracts possible adverse effects of use on human health, safety, and performance."[61]

This global emphasis on usability in the ISO standards aligns with the foundational work of Mike Cooley, an Irish engineer and workplace advocate, who coined the term "human-centered systems" in 1980 in *Architect or Bee?* He spelled out the problems in the traditional work or drafting at a drafting board with the introduction of computer-aided design. He emphasized that human-centered systems, as used in economics, computing, and design, aim to preserve or enhance human skills, in both manual and office work, in environments in which technology tends to undermine the skills that people use in their work.[62]

The framework for human-centered design relies heavily on full immersion of users in all aspects of feedback, planning, designing, and developing in order to understand the deeper impact of technology on human beings and their work. Human-centered design may more fully incorporate culturally sound, human-informed, and appropriate solutions to problems. It may improve quality by increasing the productivity of users and the operational efficiency of organizations, thus reducing training and support costs, increasing usability for people with a wider range of capabilities and therefore increasing accessibility, improving the user experience, reducing discomfort and stress, providing a competitive advantage, and contributing toward sustainability objectives.[63]

Technologists and engineers use the term "user experience" (UX) to refer to the overall experience a person has when interacting with a digital product or system, such as a website, app, software interface, or device. Its core elements are *usability, accessibility, interaction design (IxD), information architecture (IA), visual design, performance and responsiveness,* and *content.*

Usability describes how easy and intuitive a product is to use. Accessibility is about ensuring people with varying abilities can use the product. Interaction design is based on how users interact with the interface, including buttons, gestures, and responses to voice commands. The information architecture is the organization and structure of content, which impacts whether users can find what they need logically and quickly. Visual design is the aesthetics of the product, whereas performance and responsiveness focus on how fast and reliably the product responds to input. Highly usable content would be appropriately attentive to the tone, clarity, and relevance of the information presented to the user.

User experience is not an adequate framework from which to solve technology problems in the healthcare system because it focuses on a single product rather than how the system functions as a whole. Human-centered design is a better approach because it deeply considers the needs and context of users of technology from the start.

Name	Abbreviation	Concept
Human-Centered AI	HCAI	AI systems designed to align with human values
Human-Centered Design	HCD	Design methodology focusing on full systems and human needs
System Engineering for Patient Safety	SEIPS	A healthcare-specific human-centered framework
User Experience	UX	Usability of a specific product or service

Figure 2. Human-Centered Design Terminology

The advent of artificial intelligence has launched a movement to incorporate human-centered design principles into the technology (see Figure 2). Human-Centered AI (HCAI) is a methodical approach to AI system design that prioritizes human values and requirements.[64] HCAI is built on a two-dimensional framework that demonstrates the possibility of combining high levels of human control with high levels of automation. The framework positions AI as a powerful tool that empowers users rather than as an autonomous teammate.

HCAI proposes a three-level governance structure to enhance the reliability of AI systems, with the first-level software engineering teams encouraged to develop robust and dependable systems. At the second level, managers are urged to cultivate a safety culture, and at the third level, industry-wide certification establishes standards that promote trustworthy HCAI systems.

In healthcare, the lack of human-centered design in technology — from electronic health records to AI systems — has led to physician burnout, inefficiency, and poor care coordination. The high levels of burnout, physician and staff dissatisfaction with electronic health record systems, inbox agony, and all aspects of billing, coding, and prior authorization, suggest a huge need for human-centered design in healthcare to solve for the unremitting chores that have alienated clinicians and created the "moral injury" that is widely being experienced.

There is starting to be some understanding that human-centered design can help. Systems Engineering Initiative for Patient Safety (SEIPS) models are based on a human-centered design approach, which prioritizes patients' and healthcare practitioners' wants and experiences when designing systems. SEIPS 3.0 builds on earlier models by shifting the focus from isolated healthcare tasks to the entire patient journey, recognizing that effective system design must consider both clinician workflows and patient experiences across time and space. SEIPS 3.0 builds this by extending the "process" component to handle the intricacies of contemporary healthcare delivery.[65]

By putting people first, SEIPS 3.0 aims to develop healthcare systems that improve the general happiness and well-being of patients and caregivers in addition to preventing harm. The concept of the patient journey is used to describe the spatial-temporal distribution of patient interactions with multiple care settings over time. This *sociotechnical systems approach* to the patient journey and patient safety challenges designers to include the need to consider multiple perspectives, and is a response to the recognition that there are increasing challenges with care coordination for patients with chronic conditions.

SEIPS 3.0 shifts the emphasis from isolated tasks in care processes to the patient journey itself. Care process analysis focuses on healthcare delivery and the work of physicians and nurses, and asks the central question: "How can we design a patient journey that is centered on the patient and other people (e.g., caregivers, clinicians) and their needs, abilities, and constraints?" and concludes that the answer requires close attention to human-centered design, which is more than user-centered design, as other stakeholders need to be included.[66]

> "We are at a threshold moment for shaping the nature of medical care in the near and distant future. The most crucial choices confronting the medical community are not technical but ethical: the paramount fiduciary responsibility is to all humans and to the persistence of medicine as a moral and human profession."[67]

> "...the capacity for creativity depends on the very patterns in which it is embedded. In his groundbreaking 1948 paper on information theory, [Claude] Shannon cited *Finnegans Wake* as a limit case of informational density. For Shannon, Joyce's play with language showed that the amount of information in a text was a function of its departure from an expected pattern. This degree of unpredictability — Shannon called it entropy — could be measured statistically, and its quantification is foundational to machine learning (and indeed all computing). Large language models are fiction engines: they use statistics to turn randomness into information. That's not magic; it's context."[68]

Artificial intelligence is built on pattern recognition rather than an efficient and effective user experience for physicians, their staffs, and their patients. Its adaptation is inevitably a political decision, as buyers of technology determine whether to prioritize revenue generation, patent satisfaction, or clinician resilience. These are not incompatible factors; they should be multiplicative, but often their interrelatedness is not acknowledged.

These factors underscore the need for intentional design decisions about how AI will be integrated into clinical practice: Will it serve clinicians and patients, or will it primarily serve institutional metrics? The answer will shape the moral character of healthcare for decades to come.

CHAPTER 20

Human-Centered Design: Building Systems That Heal, Not Harm

Human-centered design is a discipline rooted in the belief that the best solutions arise from truly understanding the people they are meant to serve. Its methodology is organized around three key design skills: *observing, understanding*, and *creating* — each supported by practical research-based techniques drawn from ethnography, systems thinking, and creative prototyping.

Methods of observing human experience include ethnographic research through such techniques as interviewing ("fly-on-the-wall" observation and "walk-a-mile" immersion), participatory research ("what's on your radar?" and journaling), and evaluative research (heuristic review, critique, and system usability scale). The methods for developing understanding are built upon methods for analyzing challenges and opportunities with respect to people and systems, patterns and priorities, and problem framing. Methods for envisioning future possibilities include concept ideation, modeling and prototyping, and creating design rationale.[69] Design professionals have developed various techniques to learn how to better understand the people they attempt to solve problems for, which can lead to successfully implementing practical solutions. While the language of human-centered design can sound aspirational — even idealistic — it is grounded in practical, research-based methods that consistently yield effective, scalable solutions.

Human-centered design is more than a methodology — it's a philosophy rooted in empathy, collaboration, and creative problem-solving. As one leading design group frames it:

> "Embracing human-centered design means believing that all problems, even the seemingly intractable ones like poverty, gender equality, and clean water, are solvable. Moreover, it means believing that the people who face those problems every day are the ones who hold the key to their answer.

Human-centered design offers problem solvers of any stripe a chance to design with communities, to deeply understand the people they're looking to serve, to dream up scores of ideas, and to create innovative new solutions rooted in people's actual needs."[68]

However, the actual techniques used by human-centered designers are based upon proven methods for workable solutions. They emphasize that innovation is made up of three important factors: *technical, business,* and *human,* which are expressed through the lenses of *feasibility, viability, and desirability.* In healthcare, these three lenses are too often evaluated in isolation. Human-centered design insists that they must be considered together.

Human-centered design emphasizes that the focus on technology and business models is inadequate without determining its impact on the humans being served.[69] The design methods developed around products, or things, can be applied to the work environment. The work environment needs to be assessed for toxicity, as "generally toxic work environments that discourage creativity are not at all conducive to design."[70] The entire system as a whole is considered at once in human-centered design, so the framework of design moves beyond an individual product or service to focus on the entire system in which it is used.

Interaction design specifically focuses on defining the form and behavior of products, services, and systems by asking several important questions:[71]

- What tasks must the product or service support, and how?
- What workflow best enables users to achieve their goals?
- What information do users need, and when?
- What does the system need from users at each step?
- How will users transition from one task to another?
- How should features be grouped and displayed?

Paradoxically, even as clinical environments grow more complex, too little attention has been paid to designing workflows that support clinicians themselves. The result: digital tools that amplify stress rather than reduce it. Scant focus has been directed to the work environments of clinicians and their staffs as it relates to these questions, particularly as digital technologies have been added to the work environment and ever-increasing chores that are now part of the delivery system business model.

The progress that has been made in machine learning and artificial intelligence over the past decade promises unprecedented tools that can improve the lives of human beings, but also has some "dark possibilities" if it does not include human-centered artificial intelligence ways of thinking.[70] Traditional software design often stems from a rationalist mindset: structured, rule-based, and reductionist. In contrast, human-centered design is rooted in empiricism; it begins with direct observation, acknowledges complexity, and iterates through lived experience rather than rigid categories.

Rationalist thinking leads to medical information systems that require clinicians to enter reports with a limited set of categories or codes. In contrast, empiricists understand that the real world is complex, diverse, and uncertain, and tools must be refined to harness the unique gifts that human beings bring into these environments that cannot be replicated by algorithms.

At its core, human-centered design restores dignity to both patients and clinicians — dignity lost in workflows that treat people as interchangeable parts in an impersonal machine. The ubiquitous term "human-in-the-loop" still emphasizes autonomous artificial intelligence design and does not adequately acknowledge the need for ongoing human intervention, oversight, and control over technology.

While the concept of "human-in-the-loop" suggests oversight, it still centers autonomy around the machine. Human-centered AI goes further: It places people — not machines — at the heart of design, emphasizing context, care, and judgment. Human-centered artificial intelligence advocates believe that "People are not computers. Computers are not people."[71] Where "human-in-the-loop" implies occasional oversight of autonomous systems, human-centered AI insists that humans — not machines — define the goals, values, and context of every solution.

The goal of human-centric artificial intelligence design is to create products, services, and work environments that amplify, augment, empower, and enhance human performance. These systems rely on processes that extend user-experience design methods of user observation, stakeholder engagement, usability testing, iterative refinement, and continuing evaluation of human performance in the use of systems. It emphasizes human control while embedding high levels of automation.[72]

A framework based on both high levels of human control and high levels of automation is likely to produce applications that are reliable, safe, and trustworthy. Human-centered design is not anti-technology; rather, it is pro-human. In healthcare, this distinction may spell the difference between tools that heal and systems that harm (see Figure 3).

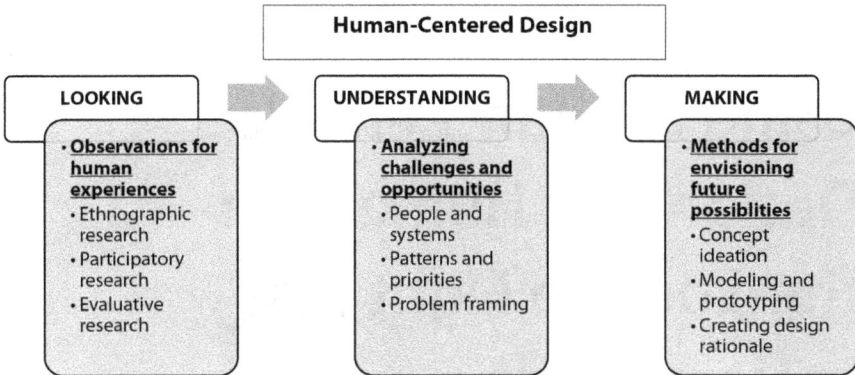

Figure 3. Elements of Human-Centered Design

Human-centered design helps us distinguish between what clinicians do best — core human care — and the chores that should be reimagined, reassigned, or automated. Only by listening deeply to those doing the work can we rebuild systems that truly support care. If we want systems that heal, not harm, then design must begin not with data or devices, but with the human beings who use them.

CHAPTER 21

Using Human-Centered Design and Humans-in-the-Loop to Fight Bias in Healthcare

This is a story about how well-intentioned care teams, absent experience and cognitive support, can be derailed by human bias, and why we need better tools rooted in human-centered design.

A few weeks ago, I received a call from my brother on a Sunday morning — a most atypical time for us to catch up. He called me as he was heading to urgent care, at the behest of his retired RN wife, because she was concerned about what he was reporting to her on a phone call while she was out of town.

My brother is a financial executive and a Marine Corps veteran of the first Gulf War, still built like a tank at age 62. He had taken a 25-mile bicycle ride on Wednesday and felt fine that evening, but woke up Thursday morning with chills, fever, lethargy, headaches, and myalgia. He made the extremely rare decision to stay home from work and tried to drink fluids, but had a poor appetite. He was no better for the next few days. On Sunday morning, he woke up with fluid retention, a six-pound weight gain, and scant brown urine.

He called his wife, who sent him to urgent care, and called me, who agreed with her recommendation. The physician in the urgent care examined him and obtained urine in the clinic, which showed 3 mg % proteinuria, no cells or casts, and brown urine with a specific gravity of 1.020. She tested him for flu and COVID, both of which were negative, and obtained a CBC and BMP and sent him home.

I had access to his patient portal and was alarmed at the proteinuria, especially in light of his acute flu-like symptoms, and waited anxiously to see the labs return. When I saw the labs, I recommended he go to the emergency room. He had a lymphocytopenia with a white count decreased at 3000, a mild thrombocytopenia, a mild hyponatremia, and mildly elevated creatinine. A repeat urine only had 150 mg % protein and remained otherwise bland.

When I saw these results, my gut instinct told me he likely had Rocky Mountain spotted fever, ehrlichiosis, or some other tick-borne illness common in the Virginia Blue Ridge Mountains this time of year, where he lives. These illnesses can be deadly so quickly so they need prompt treatment, typically with the antibiotic doxycycline. Because it takes several weeks for confirmatory tests to be obtained, it is common practice in this part of the country to treat presumptively with doxycycline while awaiting test results.

But what happened to my brother in the emergency department was a less-than-prompt diagnosis. The care team at this large, nationally acclaimed academic medical center was new in their roles. It was July, so the medical student, intern, and resident had likely not been in their roles for more than a few days. The team focused on the urine test (proteinuria), ordered a nephrology consultation, ordered a CMP, and repeated the CBC and urine test. They never, I am told, actually examined the patient. The labs were essentially unchanged, with the new information on the CMP that his liver transaminases were slightly elevated.

Although his presentation of flu-like symptoms with mild thrombocytopenia, hyponatremia, lymphopenia, mildly elevated creatinine, and mild elevated transaminases was consistent with an infectious etiology of a tick-borne virus, this diagnosis was not entertained initially, as the human cognitive bias known as anchoring bias — the tendency to rely too heavily (to "anchor") on one piece of information when making decisions (usually the first piece of information acquired) — had kicked in with the care team.

It was not until after the nephrology team had told the ER team that they did not think he needed to be admitted for his renal abnormalities that the team began to entertain any other diagnoses. Fortunately, his RN wife, MD sister (me), and DO niece (my daughter) were all aware of what was going on and refocused the team on the possibility of a tick-borne infection. He was treated with oral doxycycline and was better within 12 hours.

The cognitive biases of human beings often get in the way of evaluating all the diagnostic possibilities. Or, perhaps in the case of the care team in the emergency department that day, the inexperienced care team did not yet have the information that an experienced clinician could draw on to make a quick diagnosis.

These problems may be greatly reduced in the near future with a properly designed system. Imagine a scenario where all the information I described in the first paragraph of this story were fed into an AI engine with the ability to evaluate all the medical components of the history, physical exam, and laboratory findings, including past information from the medical record, and present a differential diagnosis up front, instantaneously, offering probabilities of diagnoses that changed over time as new information came in, and providing recommendations for further testing and treatment. The practice of medicine could look very different very quickly, allowing for more rapid and accurate diagnoses, decreasing unnecessary testing, and potentially improving the use of evidence-based clinical protocols that would lower the cost of care while enhancing its quality.

The care my brother received was not malicious nor incompetent — rather, it was anchored in a narrow interpretation of test results, disconnected from contextual reasoning. A human-centered AI, designed to learn from both patterns and the exceptions that define medicine, could have helped.

AI AND ALGORITHMIC BIAS: HOW IT ARISES

Bias in artificial intelligence is just an extension of bias in systems and data. It does not fix bias — it scales it. Human-centered, participatory design and inclusive development can provide guardrails to diminish this danger. The term "artificial intelligence" (AI) was coined by MIT professor John McCarthy, who said its purpose was to "understand and model the thought processes of humans and to design machines that mimic this behavior."[73] Large amounts of data are combined with a fast and iterative process in intelligent algorithms, which allows a machine learning system to automatically learn from patterns or features within the data.

The broad concept of artificial intelligence includes branches of algorithmic learning mechanisms such as machine learning and deep learning. *Machine learning* is a branch of AI that focuses on the study of algorithms that allow a computer program to independently perform and improve over time. *Deep learning* is a subset of machine learning that aims to reflect the function of the human brain, mimicking the human thought process.

Artificial intelligence and machine learning are founded on algorithms that human individuals create, and because humans have long held on to racial and gender biases, these biases often are unintentionally embedded in the algorithms. Once biases are within the algorithmic data, the AI will reflect these biases in its decision-making processes and task performances, which is defined as *algorithmic bias*.[74]

Key challenges remain before this ideal use of artificial intelligence in clinical decision support can be implemented. First, AI itself is based on information sources that are themselves the result of biases. Healthcare algorithms used in AI are trained on data sets that frequently lack diversity. One example of this was identified in an algorithm used to determine whether it is safe to attempt a vaginal delivery after a C-section (VBAC).[75] There are known risks associated with attempting VBAC, such as uterine rupture. In 2007, a VBAC algorithm was designed to help obstetricians assess the likelihood of safely giving birth through a vaginal delivery. The algorithm considered the woman's age, the reason for the previous C-section, race and ethnicity, and how long ago the C-section occurred.

In 2017, Vyas and colleagues[76] discovered that the original algorithm predicted that Black/African American and Hispanic/Latina women were less likely to have a successful vaginal birth after a C-section than non-Hispanic white women. This caused doctors to perform more C-sections on Black/African American and Hispanic/Latino women than on white women. In 2017, a new version of the algorithm eliminated race and ethnicity when predicting the risk of complications from VBAC, allowing doctors to make decisions based on more accurate and impartial information.

Algorithmic bias is possible in administrative tasks in healthcare as well. Consider another example of algorithmic bias in an algorithm built to determine who might need extra care in special treatment programs using a data set built on prior healthcare costs that included data from before the Affordable Care Act (ACA) was implemented.

Before the ACA, 40% of Hispanic people and 25.8% of Black people were uninsured compared to 14.8% of white people. This lack of healthcare insurance was reflected in a commercial algorithm that flagged only 17.7% of Black people as needing extra medical care, even though evidence showed that the number who would have been eligible was 46.5% had the algorithm been based on factors other than annual medical spending.[74]

In another example, an algorithm built to predict who was likely to no-show for a medical appointment was found to be flawed due to the data collection choices made by the algorithm designs; data collected included personal information such as ethnicity, financial class, and body mass index. This system excluded already marginalized groups such as Black people from low-income communities.[77]

The major challenge of algorithmic bias must be addressed before artificial intelligence can be fully integrated into clinical decision-making. The big datasets most AI algorithms need to learn from are biased due to the long history of many groups of people being absent or misrepresented in existing biomedical datasets. AI is prone to reinforcing bias, which can lead to fatal outcomes, misdiagnosis, and a lack of generalization.

According to Norori and colleagues, "Biases in healthcare can be data-driven, algorithmic, or human, and AI algorithms for healthcare can have catastrophic consequences by propagating deeply rooted societal biases. This can result in misdiagnosing certain patient groups, like gender and ethnic minorities, that have a history of being underrepresented in existing datasets, further amplifying inequalities."[78]

Some of those raising the alarm about the risks of AI propose open-science practices, including participant-centered development of AI algorithms and participatory science, responsible data sharing, and inclusive data standards to support interoperability, and code sharing, including sharing of AI algorithms that can synthesize underrepresented data to address bias.[79]

Natural language processing (NLP) began in the 1950s as an interdisciplinary field of study in artificial intelligence and linguistics. NLP uses machine learning methods that consider probabilities to generate likely language syntax. From that work in the 1980s until the present, the development of large language models has facilitated the summarization of conversations between clinician and patient into clinical notes that approximate the structure of clinical documentation and capture the foundation of medical decision-making. However, this is a long way away from utilizing AI to make clinical diagnoses. Many pitfalls must be overcome before AI can find its place in clinical decision-making:[79]

1. **Medico-legal liability:** Ultimately, it is the clinician, not the software, that is responsible for the patient's care.
2. **Reference-content reliability:** Determining the reliability of a given unit of evidence is not straightforward. Consider all the recent guidelines and recommendations that have been discovered to have been tainted by undisclosed conflicts of interest.
3. **The limited role of natural language processing and unstructured text in medical diagnosis:** It is unclear that accurate medical diagnosis/

advice mandates front-end NLP technological diagnostic systems to use structured, curated information rather than unstructured text for prioritizing diagnoses.

Artificial intelligence is not built in a vacuum, sealed off from societal realities of discrimination. Its great promise is its convenience of automated classification and discovery within large datasets, yet it may come with the downside of amplification of existing biases due to its ability to transmit bias at scale. Three types of biases can be amplified by artificial intelligence:[80]

1. **System biases:** Result from procedures and practices of particular institutions that operate in ways that result in certain social groups being favored and others disadvantaged or devalued. Institutional racism and sexism are the classic examples; other historical biases and institutional biases are equally present but less recognized. These biases are present in the datasets used in AI and in broader culture and society.

2. **Statistical and computational biases:** Result when the sample is not representative of the population. The resultant error may be due to heterogeneous data, representation of complex data in simpler mathematical representations, wrong data, and algorithmic biases such as over- and under-fitting, the treatment of outliers, data cleaning, and imputation factors.

3. **Human biases:** Reflect systematic errors in human thought based on a limited number of heuristic principles and predicting values to simpler judgmental operations, such as confirmation bias and anchoring bias, among many others.

These three types of biases can all impact AI models in unique ways, but can also be present concurrently, leading to complex biases in machine learning models. Understanding some of these biases can help us build strategies to recognize and mitigate them (see Table 3).

Technical solutionism is the increasing tendency to believe that technical solutions alone are sufficient for addressing complex problems that may have social, political, ecological, economic, and/or ethical dimensions. Unfortunately, technical solutionism is inadequate to address bias risks. It also underemphasizes human-centered design.

The McNamara Fallacy is the idea that quantitative measures are better and more objective than other observations, which leads to **techno chauvinism**. Technochauvinism is the belief that technological solutions are inherently superior to non-technological ones. **Cargo cult science** constitutes practices that superficially resemble science but do not follow the scientific method. Commentators have drawn parallels between AI and cargo cult science due to its black box interpretability, reproducibility problem, and trial-and-error processes.

The Dunning-Kruger Effect is a cognitive bias in which a person with limited knowledge in a domain may vastly overestimate their understanding of that domain. **Data dredging** is a statistical bias in which testing huge numbers of hypotheses of a dataset may appear to yield statistical significance even when the results are statistically nonsignificant.

There are types of bias that occur directly from choices made in how to normalize data based on what mathematical and statistical models are chosen for the machine learning modeling. **L1 regularization** adds bias by setting coefficients to zero, but it dramatically recues variance. **L2 regularization** adds bias by shrinking coefficients, but it balances variance without removing variables. Typically, L1 is used when you want to drop irrelevant or biased variables, while L2 modeling is used when you want stability and smoothness, to control influence without eliminating features. It is important to understand that these are mathematical choices and do not eliminate bias. Rather, they are statistical methodologies used to manage bias.

The Rashomon Effect is a term that comes from Akira Kurosaws's 1950 film "Rashomon, in which several characters witness the same crime but give mutually inconsistent testimonies. Each story reflected the individual narrator's biases, interests, and limited perspective. IN machine learning, it refers to the idea that many different models can explain the same data equally well. Which model should we trust if there are multiple explanations to fit the data set?

Artificial intelligence bias can be diminished through the processes of **TEVV (Test and Evaluation, Verification and Validation),** but remains prone to error. AI bias in healthcare has serious consequences, including misdiagnoses, unequal treatment recommendations, and exacerbation of health disparities. Several strategies can modulate AI bias in the healthcare delivery system setting.

Using a diverse and representative training set can help prevent misdiagnoses in diverse patient populations. For example, a hospital model to predict diabetes trained only on white males may fail to accurately predict these symptoms in women or minority populations. Collecting data from multiple institutions and regions and including data from underrepresented populations can help.

Bias audits and algorithmic fairness testing can become part of the routine evaluation of AI algorithms. An algorithm that predicts who should get extra care management might prioritize high healthcare spending and overlook underserved populations who underutilize care due to access issues. *Using fairness metrics and conducting regular audits* to detect and correct disparities in prediction accuracy across groups is a countermeasure.

Transparency and explainability tools guard against biases that may be embedded in treatment recommendations. Black-box AI is inadequate for clinical treatment pathways because clinicians must understand the rationale for its suggestions. Deploying explainable AI (XAI) models that provide clear reasoning for their output can reveal which features drive decisions and identify biases. Tools like SHAP (Shapley Additive exPlanations) and LIME (Local Interpretable Model-agnostic Explanations) can reveal reasoning behind black-box outputs.

Human oversight and clinical integration are crucial for ongoing patient care safety. AI systems should be designed to augment, not replace, human judgment. Including human-in-the-loop mechanisms is crucial to validating or overriding AI outputs. *Inclusive development teams* that are interdisciplinary and include data scientists, clinicians, ethicists, and representatives from marginalized groups during development and testing avoid AI models developed solely by engineers without input from clinicians or communicate with stakeholders who overlook real-world complexity.

Redefining risk and outcome variables by choosing equity-aware outcomes, such as disease burden, quality of life, or functional status, rather than economic proxies such as utilization or cost, can diminish bias to those who often receive less care. *Regulatory and ethical oversight* through the establishment of standards and certifications that require equity impact assessment and ongoing monitoring care limits vendors' release of biased AI tools into clinical use. *Community and patient engagement* in the design process can shape the design, deployment, and evaluation of AI tools in culturally competent ways.

WHY "HUMAN-IN-THE-LOOP" DESIGN MATTERS

Despite their achievement, large-language models (LLMs) are trained on large amounts of uncurated web data often scraped from internet sources with known gender, racial, cultural, and socio-economic biases. In addition, LLMs are trained in general data sets rather than those specific to healthcare.

TABLE 3. Types of Biases Impacting Large Language Models

	SYSTEMIC BIASES	STATISTICAL & COMPUTATIONAL BIASES	HUMAN BIASES
DATA SETS: Who is counted, and who is not counted?	• Issues with latent variables • Underrepresentation of marginalized groups	• Sampling and selection bias • Using proxy variables because they are easier to measure • Automation bias	• Observational bias (streetlight effect) • Availability bias (anchoring) • McNamara Fallacy
PROCESSES & HUMAN FACTORS: What is important?	• Automation of inequalities • Underrepresentation in determining utility function • Processes that favor the majority/minority • Cultural bias in the objective function (best for individuals vs. best for the group) • Reinforcement of inequalities (groups are impacted more with greater use of AI)	• Likert scale (categorical or ordinal to cardinal) • Nonlinear vs. linear • Ecological fallacy • Minimizing the L1 vs. L2 norm • General difficulty in quantifying contextual phenomena	• Groupthink leads to narrow choices • Rashomon effect leads to subjective advocacy • Difficulty in quantifying objectives may lead to McNamara Fallacy • Confirmation bias • Automation bias
TEVV: How do we know what is right?	• Predictive policing more negatively impacted • Widespread adoption of ridesharing/self-driving cars/etc. May change policies that impact the population based on use	• Lack of adequate cross-validation • Survivorship bias • Difficulty with fairness	• Confirmation bias • Automation bias

Two LLMs (ChatGPT and Claude3-Opus) were recently tested to evaluate 105,000 evidence-based medical questions and answers based on real-world physician queries. Both LLMs showed significantly inferior accuracy (Chat-GPT–55.8% and Claude3–62.4%) compared to medical professionals (82.3%) on identical questions.

More worrisome, LLM outputs varied significantly for the same prompt, raising concerns about reliability (cargo cult science!) and exhibited questionable ability to admit uncertainty despite offering this option.[81] Thus, although LLMs should continue to improve, this study highlights the three limitations of current LLMs in clinical settings: inaccurate medical information, lack of domain-specific knowledge, and unreliable output.

The National Institute of Standards and Technology contends: "AI systems are often deliberately placed into high-risk settings to counteract the known subjectivity and bias of humans. Yet considerable questions remain about how to optimally configure humans and automation. An approach to human-in-the-loop that takes into consideration the broad set of social-technical factors is necessary, especially in the context of AI bias. Human-centered design (HCD) is an approach to the design and development of a system or technology that aims to improve the ability of users to effectively and efficiently use a product. Human-centered design seeks to improve the user experience of an entire system, involving all aspects of a technology, from hardware design to software design. HCD is a methodology that has been successfully applied to a myriad of important domains. Humans and their needs drive the process, rather than having a techno-centric focus."[79]

ETHICS AND OVERSIGHT IN AI SYSTEMS

The issues related to accuracy and safety have prompted work within the domains of ethics, governance, and regulation to create guardrails for artificial intelligence in the healthcare space. Traditional artificial intelligence primarily takes on the form of predictive analytics; in contrast, generative AI is a relational AI, which is qualitatively different from predictive AI in that it creates new content, thus presenting a new range of potential ethical challenges to be addressed.[78]

In healthcare, generative AI can draft patient-portal messages, create pre-visit summaries, provide clinical summaries, and outline treatment choices for patients. The ethical framework for artificial intelligence that is applied in healthcare should ensure it is **fair, appropriate, valid, effective, and safe.**

The Belmont Report of 1979 established basic ethical principles for research involving humans: beneficence, respect for persons, and justice. These principles were subsequently applied to clinical care, with physicians held fiduciarily responsible for upholding these principles in the best interests of their patients. However, in the world of generative AI, it is sometimes difficult to evaluate whether these principles are applied. For example, LLM-generated "hallucinations," including fabricated citations, can pose an inherent risk of harm due to the probabilistic way they generate content.[82]

The four ethical principles that underlie medical practice are *justice, benefi-cence, nonmaleficence,* and *autonomy.* Any and all of these can be challenged by the black-box nature of generative AI output. The Coalition for Health AI is a public-private partnership of academics, technology companies, and the federal government that has proposed the development of a national network of health AI assurance laboratories to evaluate the safety and effec-tiveness of AI in centralized settings using representative data sets. However, such efforts have been criticized for working within a framework of "appro-priateness" rather than "beneficence," which is a stronger ethical concept.

A CALL FOR HUMAN-CENTERED AI IN CLINICAL CARE

As using AI in clinical practice begins to augment physicians' work in diag-nosing and treating conditions, determining prognosis, and improving clini-cal and administrative workflows, the technology should be "a tool guided by bioethical principles and safeguarded by human decision-making," accord-ing to Michelle McGowan, an empirical bioethicist at the Mayo Clinic.[83] She has emphasized that "as machines increase capacity to analyze data, propose diagnoses or predict treatment responses, it will be incumbent upon physi-cians to ensure that their judgment is not substituted in ways that could jeopardize patient care and introduce potential liabilities."

McGowan contends that physicians and other clinicians must address AI integrated into healthcare in the role of professional authority. Automation bias occurs when recommendations from an AI system are followed because it has been accurate in the past and requires human oversight to prevent adverse clinical outcomes. The professional role of physicians in this pro-cess may challenge traditional ways of determining bioethical approaches because of the ongoing burden of keeping up with an increasingly efficient machine-learning-enriched clinical environment. Bias in healthcare is not a new problem, but with human-centered design, we can ensure that our tools do not merely inherit our errors but help us rise above them.

Beyond the risk of algorithmic bias in artificial intelligence, an additional risk to clinical practice has become a concern for some medical ethicists: the risk of medical artificial intelligence in clinical surveillance turning clinicians into "quantified workers." Cohen and colleagues have sounded the alarm that, although AI is poised to transform medicine in ways that can improve clini-cal quality and payment processes, it also has the potential to turn clinicians into "data subjects."[84]

Ambient dictation systems can analyze speech patterns, sentiment, and con-tent such that healthcare systems could use AI scribes to assess how often clinicians' recommendations deviate from institutional guidelines. These systems could identify outliers in efficiency or performance scores based on adherence to clinical guidelines. Clinicians' communication patterns, including their responsiveness to patients, tone, or clinical reasoning, could be monitored.

Workers in other fields, including warehouse personnel and financial professionals, have already become "quantified" with AI technologies, such that their autonomy and benefits of discretionary decision-making have been replaced with protocolized behaviors. Cohen and colleagues propose a clinician's Bill of Rights for AI to prevent the loss of clinical autonomy:[84]

Right of Information: Clinicians must be informed when AI is used in a patient's care.

Right of Participation: Healthcare systems must commit to governance processes that involve clinicians in decisions about implementing AI tools that could affect their autonomy and livelihood; clinicians must have the opportunity to ask questions and express concerns about the use of AI tools without fear of retaliation.

Right of Privacy: Healthcare systems must state clearly to clinicians when and with whom AI analysis of clinician care delivery will be shared and justify sharing beyond that which is required by law or for industry self-regulation.

Right to Quality Assurance: For AI tools that may pose more than minimal risk to patients, healthcare systems must commit to pre-implementation review and regular post-implementation assessments, with results of that analysis shared with clinicians.

The emphasis on prioritizing clinician autonomy as part of a human-centered design process has the potential to enhance the promise of artificial intelligence for clinical care without worsening burnout.

Another design priority may be those aspects of clinical conversations that are considered "chit chat" and omitted in AI-generated clinical notes. As Schiff points out, the ambient listening products are built to filter out conversation that isn't relevant to the medical evaluation taking place.[85] But is "non-essential dialogue" really non-essential? The subtle nuances picked up in casual conversation with patients are often the part that drives intuition for a broader understanding of a whole-person evaluation.

As Hoff has emphasized, "there is a fight going on for the soul of health care, and primary care is at the center of the struggle." There is a competing vision between a society that wants an empathetic, highly relational care delivery system built around primary care and trusting relationships versus a more efficient, convenient, and highly transactional care delivery system built on impersonal technology and algorithms and corporations.[86]

CHAPTER 22

The Five Stages of Health Information Technology

Much of the burnout clinicians face today stems from the chore-laden workflows embedded in health IT systems — systems that evolved stage-by-stage without a unified, human-centered vision. Understanding these stages is crucial to redesigning care that puts clinicians and patients back at the center. Health information technology has developed in five stages (see Figure 4), and much of what is broken in our current healthcare system is embedded in these poorly integrated "solutions."

STAGE ONE: ADMINISTRATIVE INFRASTRUCTURE

The first stage of health information technology to reach maturity was one focused on administrative aspects of the business of medicine: billing, collecting, and scheduling. On the provider side, this technology was focused on scheduling office visits and filing claims. On the payer side, it was focused on processing claims and paying or denying them.

Electronic data exchange between providers and payers matured once technical standards that facilitated transactions between the parties were established. Health Level 7 (HL7) is a set of international standards that promote interoperability by making the sharing of healthcare data easier and more efficient across systems. Facilitating data-sharing reduces the administrative burden on providers and, thus, improves care delivery.[87]

STAGE TWO: ELECTRONIC HEALTH RECORDS

The second stage of healthcare information technology was the development of electronic health records. An electronic health record is a systematized collection of patient and population health information stored in a digital format that can be shared across different healthcare settings.

The modern origin of electronic health records dates back to the 1928 establishment of the American Association of Record Librarians (now the American Health Information Management Association) by the American

College of Surgeons in their push for standardization of medical records, but it was not until the 1960s and the development of computers that modern electronic health records emerged.

President George W. Bush called for computerized health records in his 2004 State of the Union Address, and in 2009, the American Recovery and Reinvestment Act included HITACH, which promoted the concept of meaningful use of EHRs with supported financial incentives to encourage the adoption of shared health records and the interoperability necessary to share data among providers.

Recently, Fast Healthcare Interoperability Resources (FHIR) updated HL7 standards for the exchange of resources of electronic healthcare data, designed to be flexible and adaptable so that it can be used in a wide range of settings and with a variety of healthcare information systems.

HL7 and FHIR standards allowed different systems — such as those used for billing, prescriptions, and lab results — to communicate by determining how data should be packaged and exchanged. This marked a significant leap forward in making healthcare data interoperable, although implementation remains uneven. It is easier to implement than older HL7 standards because it uses a modern web-based suite of API technology, including an HTTP-based RESTful protocol, and a choice of JSON, XML, or RDF for data representation.

STAGE THREE: POPULATION HEALTH TOOLS

With the advent of the Affordable Care Act and increasing interest in value-based care financial models, the third stage of healthcare information technology was established in the development of population health tools focused on population-level data aggregation and analytics and longitudinal, non-transactional use cases for electronic health information. These tools continue to improve, but progress is slowed by the siloes in which most healthcare data reside.

STAGE FOUR: REMOTE MONITORING AND DIGITAL TWINS

The fourth stage of healthcare information technology was built on the burgeoning technology of the Internet of Things, where multiple sources of information in the patient's home environment and ecosystem are connected directly into their healthcare delivery system. This has been manifested as "remote patient monitoring" within the healthcare industry.

Digital twinning is the process of creating a virtual replica or model of a physical object, system, or process that mirrors its real-world counterpart in real time using data, simulations, and analytics. In healthcare, a digital twin can represent anything from a specific patient's body or organ system to an entire health delivery process. As digital twinning technology becomes more adapted in the healthcare environment, it may simulate, analyze, predict, and optimize outcomes safely and efficiently at a scale that has been unprecedented.

STAGE FIVE: AI AND PREDICTIVE ANALYTICS

The fifth stage is just getting started, built on the technological capabilities of artificial intelligence and predictive analytics. Its ability to upend much of the healthcare industry through the rapid adjudication of administrative chores, exponential improvement in clinical diagnostic acumen, real-time evidence-based clinical decision support, and preemptive improvement in healthcare outcomes will be game-changing and transformative, provided the right applications and workflows are designed in human-centered ways.

Rather than evolving as an integrated whole, each layer of health IT has grown on top of legacy infrastructure. As a result, clinicians now interact with a patchwork of systems that rarely speak the same language, creating inefficiencies, frustrations, and burnout. We utilize all of these stages of health care information technologies simultaneously, and many business models are focused on solving the failings built into these less-than-mature technologies, built one on top of the other.

Stage one scheduling and revenue-cycle management technologies have been around for over half a century and are the most mature, but even so, much of the complexity of the payment system is built upon inefficient processes for payments. Electronic health records were built upon old paper-based clinical documentation, and much of the data entry duties that clinicians face now, leading to burnout, are due to the workflows that have not been maximized for human efficiency or the highest use of clinician skills.

The longitudinal technologies of stage three are even less mature because data are collected based on clinical transactions rather than longitudinal trends. Stage four remote patient monitoring is still less mature, as practitioners struggle with the question of how to make the copious data collected in real time relevant.

Each stage of HIT development brought new capabilities but also added new tasks and complexity. Without cohesive, user-driven design, these tools have burdened clinicians rather than empowered them. It is time to redesign these technologies with the user — clinician and patient alike — at the center.

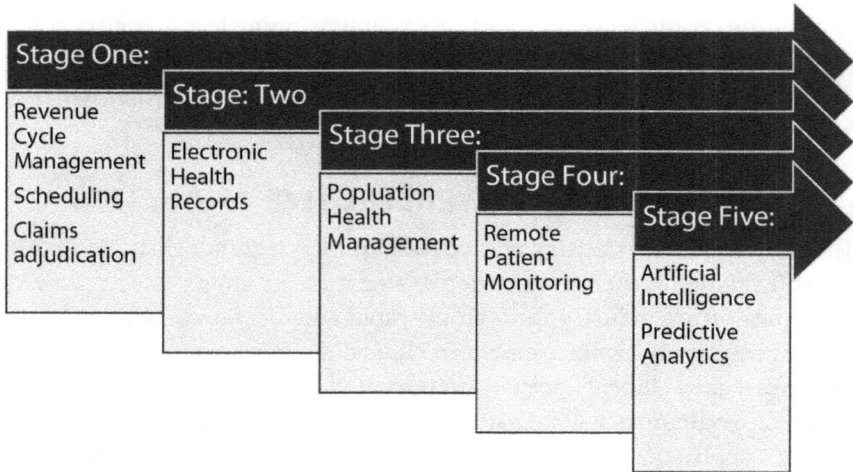

Stage One:
Revenue Cycle Management
Scheduling
Claims adjudication

Stage: Two
Electronic Health Records

Stage Three:
Popluation Health Management

Stage Four:
Remote Patient Monitoring

Stage Five:
Artificial Intelligence
Predictive Analytics

Figure 4. The Five Stages of Health Information Technology

CHAPTER 23

Design-Integrated Virtual and Digital Health

"Making sure patients get the right care, in the right place, and at the right time couldn't be a clearer set of aims."[88]

I n 2018, I was the chief executive officer of a startup company in Huntsville, Alabama, called Envision Genomics. The company focused on whole genome sequencing to diagnose rare diseases, utilizing an early AI predictive analytics technology. The technology enabled nearly instantaneous diagnoses of rare diseases that previously took on average eight or more years and more than $250,000 to diagnose. The company ultimately failed as a business for a number of reasons, including the reluctance of the conservative insurance industry to reimburse for the associated diagnostic testing, despite its financial and clinical benefits.

Although it is easier to get these tests reimbursed by insurance in 2025, many companies require less expensive but also less definitive diagnostic testing prior to paying for the definitive test. There is a significant need in healthcare to redesign the diagnostic process based on the efficiencies of new technologies and to incorporate cost-effective diagnostic pathways that eliminate unnecessary testing.

TRANSACTIONAL TELEHEALTH AND THE "JOBS TO BE DONE"

An equally important need is to redesign how individuals access the healthcare services they need. While Envision Genomics was winding down, I supplemented my income by working for a national telehealth company for several months. I performed over 5,000 telehealth clinical interactions in a nine-month period for patients in Alabama and North Carolina, where I had medical licenses.

This work was pre-pandemic, and telehealth was not yet widely used. I learned from that experience that a significant number of well-insured patients preferred interactions through telehealth with a physician they did not know rather than interacting with a primary care or specialist physician with whom they had an established relationship. The benefit of telehealth was based on its availability 24 hours a day, with no waiting.

What I learned from the experience has significantly shaped my understanding of how the chores of healthcare can be designed out of the system. In contrast to my personal internal medicine practice, where I had extensive medical knowledge of the patients' prior history in the copious electronic medical records, the telehealth company had designed an electronic health record that was far more efficient to use, and typically, the patient transactions were fast and satisfactory.

Patients seeking care via telehealth do so, or did so pre-pandemic, for purely transactional reasons. Typically, they had simple medical problems for which they did not want to take time off work to go to a physician's office, an urgent care, or the emergency room. Almost always, they were correct that the problems they were calling about could easily be handled without a face-to-face in-person interaction.

Much of what they wanted was treatment for allergies, upper respiratory infections, urinary tract infections, conjunctivitis, gout, low back pain, shingles, rashes, dental pain, and various musculoskeletal conditions. When it was clear that the caller was experiencing a true emergency, such as cardiac chest pain, a system was set up with nurse triage to call an ambulance and stay on the line with the caller until emergency care could be rendered.

More often than not, I was able to accurately diagnose and provide evidence-based medical care. The telehealth company provided almost immediate feedback with respect to my prescribing habits and patient satisfaction scores, and the medical director let me know relatively quickly if I was not following their guidelines for specific conditions.

The electronic record I used for the telehealth was proprietary for them and the easiest I have ever used. I used it on my iPad, and it was fast, easy, and with minimal unnecessary clicks. The patient's demographic information was easily displayed along with self-reported allergies, meds, any prior telehealth company transactions, and a review of systems and patient-reported symptoms. The symptom-specific templates were fantastic, and I was able to document accurately and close a note typically within two minutes of the end of a transaction. Translation services were available, as were three-way interactions with family members for patients with dementia or other special needs.

The clinical documentation was easy, and the coding and billing were not part of my workflow at all. The contrast between this intuitive, chore-free telehealth EHR and the more burdensome traditional EHRs I have used illustrates how thoughtful design can liberate clinicians from unnecessary work.

Clay Christensen taught us that the "jobs to be done" that a consumer "hires" a product or service for often differ from the seller's intended use.[31] The patients who used my services on telehealth often sought care not just for convenience, but for privacy, autonomy, and relief from systemic friction. For example, an astonishing number of people wanted a prescription for anti-smoking medications such as varenicline or bupropion. They wanted to try it on their own without interacting with their primary care physician.

Likewise, for example, a surprising number of individuals requested treatment for genital herpes simplex via telehealth because they did not want their personal physician to know. Many individuals needed a month's supply of their chronic medications because they could not get a refill from their primary care physician without an appointment, and their physician had no appointments available. For telehealth patients, the jobs to be done center around patient preferences, privacy, and access.

TELEHEALTH TRANSFORMATION DURING COVID

My telehealth experience was pre-pandemic, and Medicare and many commercial payers at the time did not pay for telehealth services, so it was not yet a primary way patients accessed medical services. The business model for the telehealth companies was in large part based on an add-on benefit for the employer-based insurance market, which saw the benefit of lower costs for virtual access for employees in contrast to paying for days off work and emergency room and urgent care visits.

By the time the pandemic hit in the winter of 2020, I was chief executive of Eventus WholeHealth, a company that focuses on an integrated primary care and mental health model for medically vulnerable adults who reside in nursing homes, assisted living facilities, or are homebound due to their frailty. Like the rest of the healthcare world, when CMS allowed televisits, we rapidly changed our business model from being face-to-face transactions in the home, skilled nursing facility, or assisted living setting to telehealth visits, when at all possible. Our company spanned five states at the time, yet we were able to provide access to essential services with tele-technology nearly overnight, once issues such as a lack of Wi-Fi in many facilities were overcome, and nurses in the facilities were trained to help with the video technology. COVID changed patient expectations with respect to access; many accepted televisits for the first time, and many more discovered the benefits of using portals to communicate with their physicians' practices.

POST-PANDEMIC REGRESSION AND FUTURE POTENTIAL

After the pandemic, many practices returned to offering a minimal number of televisits, despite more open payment for the services. One of the reasons was that the traditional electronic health records were not built to make televisits the easy-peasy experience I had with the telehealth company. It became one more set of one thousand clicks in the enterprise-wide electronic health record.

Additionally, physicians had a lot of ambulatory clinical space that needed to be filled with patients due to real estate overhead costs. In the future, physicians may need half the space or have twice the number of physicians using the space, with some working from home doing televisits follow-ups and some in the office seeing patients in person. As the chores of medicine are re-examined, including what absolutely has to be done in person versus what does not, healthcare can become far more efficient. I imagine a future healthcare delivery system where integrated virtual and digital health becomes a real digital front door into an efficient healthcare delivery system, rather than an inefficient inbox nightmare for the clinical staff that it is today.

What we have learned is that convenience, efficiency, and discretion matter deeply to patients. Virtual and digital care, if thoughtfully integrated and designed around human needs — not billing systems or institutional inertia — can become the foundation for a truly responsive, modern healthcare system. Now that we have all experienced the rapid changes and regressions of the COVID and post-COVID world, there is a significant opportunity to use human-centered design principles for healthcare system improvements.

During COVID, clinicians were often left out of virtual care workflow design, leading to inefficient, "bolt-on" telehealth systems and a regression to pre-COVID workflows. Virtual care workflow design could be co-designed with frontline clinicians and patients using the human-centered design principle of involving users early and continuously.

During the pandemic lockdowns, elderly patients in SNFs and rural patients often lacked internet access due to infrastructure limitations or limited technology literacy. Designing for inclusivity by using the human-centered design principle of designing for "edge cases" would address outliers and barriers.

We faced this challenge at Eventus WholeHealth and deployed tech-trained staff to assist with the calls and hotspot technology tools. During the pandemic, pop-up vaccine clinics in underserved neighborhoods were successful not because of apps or portals, but because teams coordinated across community groups, designing on-the-ground logistics around people's real lives with after-hours and weekend hours, no appointment required. This focused on the principle of human-centered design of adapting systems to human contexts, not the other way around.

CHAPTER 24

From Vision to Action: Strategy, Tactics, and the Future of Healthcare

The U.S. healthcare system resembles organized chaos. This book explores how that chaos can be untangled by distinguishing between what is truly essential to patient care and what are merely chores.

But identifying the problem is only the beginning. Designing a better system requires clarity in process, beginning with strategy, followed by tactics, and then execution. Once that is complete, redesigning the system to eliminate chores requires very specific processes that are thought through and enacted in a particular order. Strategy precedes tactics, and execution requires the stepped implementation of basic measures.

Everyone has a default future, the one that unfolds if we let events play out without intervention. But we can rewrite that future. Visioning an alternative future is the first step. Yet a vision without a strategy is just a hallucination. Strategy is not a hope, an aspiration, or a goal. It solves real problems. Physicians, in fact, are well trained in strategic thinking. A good clinician makes an accurate diagnosis, adopts a guiding policy (evidence-based medicine), applies a coherent sequence of interventions, evaluates and mitigates risks, and leverages proven advantages — just as a good strategist does.

We make accurate diagnoses by applying our clinical training to the art of taking a history, performing a physical examination, and doing appropriate diagnostic testing. Evidence-based medicine and clinical protocols are our guiding policies. A strategy without leadership will fail.

The orders and delivery of treatment for a condition such as diabetic ketoacidosis is an example of a coherent administration of tactics. The conversation a urologist has with a patient about the risks and benefits of surgery versus watchful waiting for early-stage prostate cancer in a shared decision-making process is an example of how we focus on risks and how to mitigate them.

The early treatment of rheumatoid arthritis with DMARDs (disease-modifying antirheumatic drugs) greatly improves outcomes and is one example of how we understand the competitive advantage of one tactic in what used to be a much worse prognosis. In a similar manner, we need to apply these tactics in addressing the ongoing problems in our healthcare delivery system.

Physicians are natural strategists. The way they approach patient care — diagnosing, planning, treating, and adjusting — mirrors the strategic mindset we must bring to healthcare system transformation. Table 4 illustrates the correlation between clinical practice and strategic execution.

TABLE 4. Physicians as Natural Strategists

CLINICAL PRACTICE	STRATEGIC EXECUTION
Diagnose the problem.	Make an accurate diagnosis of the systemic issue.
Use clinical guidelines or protocols.	Apply a guiding policy to address the challenge.
Prescribe a treatment plan.	Execute a coherent sequence of tactics.
Manage side effects and risks.	Mitigate risks through planning and shared decision-making.
Choose targeted, effective therapies early.	Leverage competitive advantage through early, high-impact actions.

Here is what we healthcare leaders need to do together:

• **Partner** across organizations to reduce clinical variation and cost and accelerate consumer-focused value.
• **Build** a culture of transparency, trust, teamwork, and problem-solving.
• **Redesign** business models. If the task doesn't require a clinician, it shouldn't be done by a clinician; if it doesn't require in-person care, it shouldn't happen in person.
• **Learn** together using predictive analytics, precision medicine, and micro-segmentation to match interventions to patient needs.

The following strategic readiness checklist can help you determine if your organization is ready to turn vision into action:

STRATEGIC READINESS CHECKLIST
Vision & Execution
• Are we moving fast enough?
• Do we know our capability gaps and how to close them?
• Are we playing offense or defense?

Patient-Centered Focus

- Is the patient truly at the center of our efforts?
- Have we identified and eliminated unnecessary chores in health-care?
- Are we aligning with consumer preferences and access needs?

Design & Technology

- Are we using human-centered design in our solutions?
- Do we know when a human must be in the loop — and which human?
- Are we applying AI ethically and strategically?

Culture & Communication

- Is radical communication planning embedded in our execution?
- Does our culture reflect our stated mission, vision, and values?

Strategy without action is theory. Tactics without strategy is chaos. If we are to build the future our patients deserve, we must unite vision with execution, starting now.

CHAPTER 25

It's Moral Injury, not Burnout

The staggering rates of clinician burnout mask a deeper truth. Burnout is not just a workplace epidemic; it is a signal of a deeper crisis: moral injury. Moral injury is not a failure of personal resilience but a breach between professional values and systemic realities. Moral injury occurs when healthcare professionals are unable to provide the care they believe is right, often due to systemic barriers beyond their control. The injury occurs when clinicians are forced to act in ways that violate their ethical commitments, leading to guilt, anger, and a crisis of purpose (see Table 5).

Burnout is defined by emotional exhaustion, depersonalization, and a diminished sense of accomplishment. These symptoms signal psychological harm, but they originate from external conditions — inefficiencies, misaligned incentives, and ethical dissonance — not personal weakness.[89] The astonishing statistics on physician burnout indicate that half of physicians and two-thirds of nurses in the country reported symptoms of burnout in 2023.[90]

The exhaustion that signals burnout encourages clinicians to distance themselves emotionally and cognitively from their work. Emotional exhaustion depletes a healthcare provider's capacity to be involved with and responsive to the needs of patients, and depersonalization puts a distance between clinicians and the patients they serve by ignoring the qualities that make them unique and engaging people. Burned-out clinicians cannot effectively serve their patients, which significantly affects patient outcomes, staff turnover, and the sustainability of the clinician workforce.

But burnout is a symptom, and labeling a clinician as burned out puts the blame on the individual rather than the system that creates the symptoms. As Zubin Damania (aka ZDoggMD) makes clear, "burnout" is a form of victim-shaming. He explains:[91]

> "It's saying you're not resourceful enough, you're not resilient enough, you're not strong enough to adapt to a system," he says. "Humans are moral idealistic creatures that resonate love for other humans. And what happens when our moral ideals meet the real world where we cannot give our patient the care, we know that we could give if we had the tools and the resources and the autonomy to do it? What happens when we're trained in our schooling

to give the best possible care to patients regardless of their socioeconomic status, regardless of their race, regardless of their condition or their gender? ...then we meet the real world where it's all about the insurance company's bottom line, it's all about the hospital system's revenue. What happens when a moralistic clinician encounters a system which goes against their values, makes them feel disrespected and powerless? This is not burnout; this is moral injury."

Over the years, I've encountered deeply unsettling examples of profit-driven decisions that betray our mission as healers:

A chief financial officer of a large, highly profitable hospital system with a nationally recognized children's hospital told me he was not interested in hearing about a program that uses whole-genome sequencing to diagnose and treat rare diseases in children early, because it would decrease their hospital cases.

An executive in the nursing home industry told me he was opposed to vaccine mandates for staff during the epidemic because it would decrease the number of staff available to take care of the elderly, frail patients in the facilities he was managing, and would decrease the facility's profits.

A physician told me he opposed vaccination during COVID because he thought it better to "just let all the old people die from it."

I have spent hours on hold with a payer attempting to get prior approval for a breast MRI for a patient who carried the BRCA gene and had watched her sisters and mother all die from breast cancer. The prior authorization system was designed by that payer to be difficult and expensive for physicians to use.

These are not isolated incidents; they are symptomatic of a system in which financial incentives often override clinical judgment and human dignity. My colleagues all have similar stories. When we continue to fight the good fight for our patients, and impossible barriers are placed that prevent the best possible care, it is no wonder we feel emotionally exhausted and depersonalized and become less effective at performing our mission-focused professional roles.

Psychiatrist Jonathan Shay coined the term "moral injury" in 1994 during his work with soldiers and veterans to describe their psychological distress in participating in actions that violated their deeply held moral beliefs.[92] Since then, the concept of moral injury has expanded to describe similar types of psychological distress experienced by healthcare professionals who must make life-or-death decisions or take actions that conflict with their morals and beliefs. Examples include having to prioritize limited resources to the detriment of care for some patients, witnessing death and injury on a large scale, or participating in actions based on institutional policies that conflict with best care for patients.

During the COVID-19 pandemic, healthcare workers experienced moral injury on a massive scale, as they faced difficult decisions regarding patient care in extremely challenging circumstances and with very little strategic control. When clinicians are forced to spend their days fighting unnecessary battles — prior authorizations, bureaucratic delays, poorly designed EHRs — they are pushed further from their core mission. These chores aren't just inefficient; they are morally corrosive.

Although the root cause of moral injury in healthcare is often attributed to financialized business models that prioritize the bottom line rather than good patient care, moral injury is also widely reported among physicians who practice in publicly funded healthcare systems in the United Kingdom and Europe. Given its widespread presence across the global health workforce, its etiology can be broadened from a focus on a specific financial model to the chronic and systemic healthcare system failure in which demands are placed on healthcare professionals far in excess of the resources and support available to them.

One proposed theoretical framework for addressing moral injury is based on three interventions:[93]

1. **Individual interventions:** Improving personal skills and resilience of healthcare professionals.
2. **Organizational interventions:** Reducing sources of stress and moral injury in the work environment.
3. **Societal and structural interventions:** Implementing policy reforms and public health initiatives and influencing societal shifts in how healthcare work is valued and supported.

One error in addressing moral injury is focusing only on the individual's response to stress, on the need for "grit" or "resilience." The origins of moral injury are at the environmental and system level, and solutions need to be systemic in nature. As Jenny Byrne argues in her study of moral injury, just as the Cherokee link the health of the individual to the health of the community with a concern about "soul injury," the focus on burnout and resilience misses the mark.[94] Moral injury resolves with system reform. Understanding this within the context of "core versus chore" facilitates a reengineered, healthy work environment.

Some specific strategies that organizations can deploy at the system level to decrease symptoms of moral injury and its consequential burnout behaviors are:

1. Foster open communication where healthcare professionals can speak about their challenging experiences and moral dilemmas, and where confidential reporting systems exist free from fear of retribution.
2. Provide mental health support within the context of acknowledging the psychological impact of moral injury.
3. Provide ethical training and education to guide professional teams through complex moral decisions.
4. Enact policy and systemic changes that address the origins of moral injury and reduce administrative burdens to improve the focus on patient-centered care and ensure adequate staffing to reduce overwork and burnout.
5. Create safe spaces for breaks and rest.
6. Encourage advocacy and empowerment through participation in leadership opportunities and advocacy groups.

Systems thinking, rather than the focus on the injured individual, is how moral injury and burnout are resolved. A paradigm shift that evaluates systemic dysfunction moves away from traditional remedies such as resilience training, mindfulness, and therapy to ask the important question: What aspects of the system create the conditions for moral injury or burnout? Within that context, system-level solutions can be designed, specifically focused on human-centered design principles.

TABLE 5. Burnout vs. Moral Injury: What's the Difference?

BURNOUT	MORAL INJURY
Symptom	Root cause
Individual failure	System betrayal
Treated with resilience training	Requires system redesign
Emotional exhaustion	Ethical conflict
Focus: Self-care	Focus: Structural reform

A system-level solution to moral injury can be approached through human-centered design:

1. *Empathize with Users:* **Understand the lived experience of clinicians and create space for emotional truth.**

- Foster open communication where healthcare professionals can speak about moral dilemmas without fear of retribution.
- Provide mental health support that acknowledges the psychological toll of moral injury.
- Create safe spaces for breaks, rest, and reflection.

2. *Define the Problem Clearly:* **Recognize that the issue lies in the environment, not the individual.**
   - Shift the narrative from "burnout" to "moral injury" to correctly identify root causes.
   - Provide ethical training to support teams facing complex moral decisions.
   - Use data to identify when systemic pressures lead to recurring ethical compromise.

3. *Brainstorm and Co-Design with Frontline Users:* **Involve clinicians in reimagining workflows, policies, and environments.**
   - Encourage advocacy and empowerment through leadership and system redesign roles.
   - Promote confidential reporting systems that elevate issues to decision-makers.
   - Use interdisciplinary design teams (clinicians + IT + admin) to reimagine burdensome processes.

4. *Prototype and Test Organizational Change:* **Make iterative improvements to system-level policies and environments.**
   - Enact policy changes that reduce administrative burdens and reinforce patient-centered care.
   - Ensure adequate staffing to prevent overload and task saturation.
   - Pilot task redistribution (e.g., removing non-core chores from clinician workflows) and refine based on clinician feedback.

5. *Implement and Evaluate at Scale:* **Sustain change by embedding human-centered metrics and feedback loops.**
   - Embed metrics of moral well-being and ethical alignment into organizational dashboards.
   - Build continuous improvement into workflows with regular feedback from frontline clinicians.
   - Align organizational culture with mission and values — where healing professionals feel respected and empowered.

A hidden toll of moral injury is the culture of silence that surrounds it. When clinicians feel they cannot voice ethical concerns without fear of retaliation, the trauma compounds. Normalizing discussion of moral distress must be a core design objective of any reformed system. As artificial intelligence, digital health, and virtual care redefine how medicine is delivered, we stand at a pivotal crossroads. We can use these tools to depersonalize care further, or to humanize it more than ever before. Recognizing moral injury as a system design flaw gives us the blueprint for the latter. It invites us to redesign healthcare in ways that honor both our patients and us. And doing so allows us to reclaim the meaning and purpose at the heart of medicine.

CHAPTER 26

Burnout Is Gendered: The Disproportionate Toll on Women Physicians

Physician burnout affects doctors across all specialties and demographics, but it does not do so equally. Research consistently shows that female physicians experience significantly higher rates of burnout than their male counterparts.

This gender gap is not due to inherent personal differences but reflects a systemic set of inequities baked into the design of healthcare delivery. The drivers are multifactorial and include structural, cultural, and interpersonal dynamics, as outlined below:[95]

1. **Differences in resources**: Women typically have less staff support, less financial support, and experience disparities in mentoring and sponsorship.
2. **Higher workloads**: Women spend more time on average per patient, more time in the electronic health record, have more messages from patients and staff, and experience higher emotional demands from patients.
3. **Challenges in work-life integration**: Women experience disproportionate outside responsibilities compared to men, including childcare and care for older parents, and insufficient support related to pregnancy and parental leave.
4. **Barriers to meaning at work**: Women report less professional fulfillment than their male colleagues, lower self-compassion, and lower perceived appreciation from their teammates and patients.
5. **Less autonomy**: report less control over their workload and schedules, and insufficient time to see patients during office visits.
6. **Organizational culture factors**: There is a lack of women in leadership roles, especially those with decision-making and budgetary authority, compensation disparities across all specialties, fewer career advancement

opportunities, lower rates of academic promotion, gender bias, microaggressions, and harassment, and bias against physician mothers.

7. **Threats to social support and community**: Women experience microaggressions from patients, colleagues, and staff, have higher rates of imposter syndrome, and have significant professional isolation in certain subspecialties.

I have written about this elsewhere,[96] but I want to emphasize here a few aspects that were not core to the themes in my previous book. First, much of today's healthcare work environment was designed during a time when the physician workforce was predominantly male and supported by partners who managed domestic responsibilities. These outdated assumptions fail to accommodate the dual roles many women now navigate — professional and caregiving — leading to high levels of burnout and structural system strain.

The prolonged years of residency training programs often overlapped with women's maximum fertility and child-rearing years, encouraging women to choose primary care specialties rather than the more lucrative procedural specialties, long and still the purview of male physicians ... and, perhaps, also more highly paid *because* they are the purview of male physicians.

In outpatient settings, female physicians report needing 26% more time per patient than allotted, compared to 21% more time for male physicians — yet schedules rarely reflect this difference. They also care for more patients with complex psychosocial needs, write longer notes, and receive more EHR messages.

Compared with male physicians, female physicians have more patients with complex psychosocial problems. The greater amount of time on average female physicians spend with their patients results in, on average, a $22,000 lower mean income than that of men. Women have 1.6 times the odds of reporting burnout compared with men.[97] Overall, 64% of women physicians defer important life decisions, such as getting married or having children, in pursuit of their medical career.[98]

Patients have differing expectations of female versus male physicians. Female patients tend to seek more empathic listening and longer visits, especially with female physicians; however, female doctors are not allotted more time for this. Female doctors have more female patients than male doctors, and more patients with psychosocial complexity.[99] Female physicians experience significantly more patient-initiated messages and electronic health record workload despite an equivalent number of results and panel size.[100]

Female surgeons spend more time documenting patient encounters, write longer notes, and spend more time in the EHR system compared with male surgeons.[101] In this context, the chores of healthcare — documentation, EHR messaging, patient emotional labor — are not only more frequent for women but are expected and culturally invisible. These are unacknowledged tasks that disproportionately erode well-being. The cumulative weight of longer visits, increased EHR demands, and more complex patients creates a compounding burden on female physicians — one that rarely maps to formal job descriptions or scheduling algorithms.

Notably, studies have shown that patients treated by female physicians experience lower mortality and hospital readmission rates — suggesting that what we currently undervalue in workflows may, in fact, improve outcomes.

Women clearly work in different ways than men performing similar roles in healthcare, with different performance expectations from their patients as a result, leading to higher levels of burnout. In addition, the increased expectations of other gendered roles, such as greater child and eldercare responsibilities, more household chores, such as meal preparation, are a natural setup for the quantitative increases in burnout identified in women compared to men. Therefore, redesign of clinical workflows that reduces clinical documentation burden will have an outsized impact on female physicians compared to male physicians.

Currently, 55% of medical students are female — the third year in a row in which women have made up the majority of medical school students, applicants, and matriculants. Solving for the chores in healthcare will have an outsized strategic advantage for those organizations that understand the strategic advantage of solving for gender bias at the chore level of healthcare.

Redesigning clinical workflows to eliminate low-value tasks and reducing documentation burden is not just a matter of equity; it's a strategic imperative. Health systems that fail to address gendered chore burdens risk accelerating burnout, talent loss, and reduced patient satisfaction — undermining care quality and organizational sustainability. Organizations that proactively address gendered burnout will not only retain top talent but will also gain a competitive edge in a rapidly evolving workforce.

By considering the outsized impact of burnout on women in the healthcare delivery system, we can redesign the working environment for sustainability and improved outcomes. Lombarts and Verghese emphasized recognizing gender bias is not to create a "battle of the sexes." Rather, "every physician's effort is needed to provide the best care." Human-centered design thinking can help with these efforts.[102]

Lombarts and Verghese point out that traditionally "masculine" endowments still largely define how medicine is currently organized and practiced, emphasizing "protocolized medicine, measurement practices, systems-based thinking, efficiency, and authoritarian leadership" while deemphasizing "traditionally female-coded qualities" such as "nurturance, intuition, communality, and expressiveness." They worry that today's advances in artificial intelligence will "further consolidate the culturally coded 'masculine' view and marginalize the 'soft skills' even further."

The application of human-centered design principles in the design of AI-augmented workflows can help transcend the limitations of gendered cultural constructs so that patient-centeredness, empathy, and communication are integrated into the healthcare environment. Human-centered design asks: *Who is this system serving?* and *Whose pain points are invisible in existing workflows?* By centering female physicians in workflow redesign — gathering ethnographic data, mapping their journeys, and co-developing solutions — we can create environments that recognize, value, and support the distinct contributions they bring to care. By addressing the gendered nature of chore burden through thoughtful, inclusive design, we realign our health system with its core purpose: to heal — sustainably, equitably, and humanely.

CHAPTER 27

Redesigning Healthcare's Financial Engine: Solving the Hidden Drivers of Dysfunction

ehind the scenes of every clinic visit or hospital stay is a complex financial ecosystem that shapes how, when, and why care is delivered. Understanding this financial scaffolding is key to eliminating the inefficiencies — the "chores" — that burden clinicians and patients alike.

All businesses are made up of the same components: people, processes, technologies, capital resources, and culture. When people can acquire resources to supply goods or services that others find valuable, a business is born. The way people interact with one another and with their customers and other stakeholders comprises the culture. The resources are funded by capital.

WHAT IS CAPITAL AND WHY DOES IT MATTER?

Capital, simply put, is any resource used to produce value in the economy, whether a physical asset such as a building or equipment, an intangible asset such as intellectual property, technological innovations, human capital (people), or cultural capital. Financial capital most commonly refers to the money a business uses to either meet upcoming expenses or to invest in new assets and projects.

Understanding how the money flows in the complex healthcare market creates opportunities to eliminate many of the inefficient "chores" of providing healthcare.

The financial complexity of the healthcare industry stems from the fact that providing healthcare services is expensive due to the need for substantial resources in people and technology. In addition, the need for healthcare is intermittent when it comes to high-intensity services such as surgeries, hospitalizations, and treatment for complex illnesses. Although most people will need such services at some time in their lives, for the most part, these needs are intermittent and unpredictable with respect to time and duration.

At the beginning of the 20th century, the average life expectancy was 47 years, and clinical care needs were mostly related to acute, mostly infectious illnesses. By 1950, life expectancy had increased to 68 years, with an increasing need to treat some chronic diseases, such as cardiovascular diseases and cancer. By the beginning of the 21st century, life expectancy had increased to 77 years on average, with the cost of chronic diseases exceeding acute illnesses.

By 2050, preventative care and precision medicine may dominate healthcare costs, and life expectancy may increase even more, but the financing will need to be simplified from the current cross-subsidization that no longer meets the needs of the public at large.

THE ORIGINS OF INSURANCE AND WHY IT NO LONGER FITS

Healthcare's financial model was established before the potentially catastrophic costs of healthcare services were realized. Physicians provided healthcare in a "fee-for-service" model and typically charged based on the patient's ability to pay. However, as technological advances in treatments required highly intensive resource development, the cost of healthcare exceeded the ability of individuals living paycheck to paycheck to pay. Options include taxation with governmental payment for services as they were needed, which is the predominant method of financing healthcare in many developed countries, or an insurance market, which is the model that developed in the United States.

Insurance is a hedge against a rare event. One pools one's resources with others to be covered for an unlikely event, such as a house fire, knowing that at the population level, some people will experience a house fire, and if enough people pay a little bit to prevent the catastrophic impact of being the one who experiences it, then everyone who buys the insurance will be better off. The concept embedded in these insurance models is that you expect to never have to use the insurance, but do not want the risk that such a catastrophic event might occur.

Traditional healthcare insurance developed when the likelihood of a catastrophic healthcare event, like requiring surgery or hospitalization, was rare. But now, the health insurance industry prefers to call it a "health plan" rather than "health insurance" because it covers most types of health services and everyone expects to use it.

The first health insurance did not cover physician services, which were relatively inexpensive, but acute hospitalization. However, over time, health insurance morphed from being something that covered occasional expensive services to something that is comprehensive in coverage for acute needs like hospitalizations, physician services, medications, and other clinical services. The result is a highly complex system of multiple payers with multiple payment rules and numerous tasks for healthcare providers seeking payment for the services they provide. The cross-subsidization of healthcare expenses creates additional administrative complexity. Overutilization of profitable services induces managed care and regulatory complexity as a countermeasure.

THE HIDDEN COSTS OF COMPLEXITY

When those who receive healthcare services are not those who directly pay for them, there is a disconnect between the interest of the payer, who wants to pay only for what is either regulatorily necessary or medically necessary, and the patient, who wants as much service as possible that they believe would benefit them.

This disconnect is called "moral hazard" in the insurance industry. Moral hazard is an economic term describing a situation in which someone takes more risks because they believe another party will cover the costs. In the case of a house fire, someone with homeowners' insurance may not be as diligent about preventing a fire. In the case of healthcare, someone may live an unhealthier life or may focus on overutilization of services that they wouldn't use if they had to pay for them directly.

For healthcare services provided by governmental payers, these natural conflicts are managed with regulatory mandates regarding covered services, a focus on preventing fraud and abuse for those receiving unnecessary care, and political policy work regarding what services are covered and for whom.

Countries with universal healthcare typically set national budgets for healthcare expenditures. For those of us in systems where the payer is our employer or we are paying for benefits established by a healthcare insurer, "managed care" becomes the tool by which this moral hazard is navigated. Our benefits are defined by the healthcare policy we either purchase directly or that our employer provides for us.

Even in this "private" setting, healthcare policy is highly regulated. The National Committee for Quality Assurance (NCQA) developed the HEDIS

(Health Effectiveness Data and Information Set) performance tool that more than 90% of health plans use to measure performance on important dimensions of care and service, including preventative screening, chronic disease management, access to care, patient satisfaction, and behavioral health.

The HEDIS criteria are mandated by CMS for Medicare Advantage and Medicaid managed care plans. Self-funded health plans offered by employers are governed by ERISA (Employee Retirement Income Security Act of 1974), which sets a minimum standard for most employer-sponsored benefit plans and is enforced by the U.S. Department of Labor. The Affordable Care Act regulated many other aspects of private healthcare insurance.

So how healthcare is paid for is extremely complex in the United States, where federal programs such as Medicare and Medicare intersect with employer-covered insurance, both self-funded and fully-insured, private Medicare and Medicaid plans, military and veterans benefits, the perennially underfunded public health system, and, increasingly, an alternative pseudo-insurance market developing among certain religious groups dissatisfied with governmentally mandated benefits in the legitimate health care market.

The administrative complexity of understanding the regulations, benefits, and rules of this highly fragmented system underlies much of the "chores" inherent in our current healthcare ecosystem. When physicians must navigate 30 payers with 30 different preauthorization rules to deliver one treatment, we've turned caregiving into paperwork. Healthcare's financial inefficiency doesn't just waste money — it consumes clinicians.

THE MANY FACES OF CAPITAL

On the other side of the table are the sources of capital that healthcare businesses access to provide goods and services to the market. There are only a few ways for businesses to acquire capital: use assets they already have, such as cash on hand (a liquid asset), sell an asset (land, property, equipment, a business unit) to convert it into a liquid asset, or get the capital from someone else through a loan, investment in the company, or as a grant or charitable contribution.

Traditionally, medical groups owned by physicians had a hard time accessing many sources of capital because they are set up as for-profit professional companies that, by law, cannot be owned by non-physicians. Consequently, physician groups were reliant either on their own assets and resources or bank loans. Health systems that are set up as not-for-profit are exempt from taxes and have access to the bond markets. Those set up as for-profit have access to both public markets and private equity capital. For any and all sources of capital, it is important to understand the business models of the capital markets themselves in order to understand the impact on one's own business.

Bank Loans: Traditionally, commercial loans were the sole source of funding for physician-owned medical practices, and often the collateral used to cover the risk of the loan was personal assets, such as one's home. For this reason, many physicians also invested in the real estate in which their practices were housed, as the physical asset of real estate allowed them the ability to finance practice loans and build equity in the real estate over time.

As the cost of medical education has increased, so has the amount of student loan debt physicians hold; their ability to access bank loans has diminished, especially for primary care physicians.

Private Equity: Over the past couple of decades, private equity has exploded across the United States' economic landscape as a result of regulatory changes that allowed private sources of equity to be utilized for riskier investments than traditional bank loans could manage. Private equity has sponsored much of the technological innovation that has occurred over the past 30 years and is now firmly embedded in the economic fabric of most industries in the United States. Understanding the nuances of how the equity market is organized is important to understanding its impact on the healthcare industry.

Typically, for new businesses, individuals must come up with the initial capital from personal sources or what may be called a "friends and family" round of early equity investment before the business has a proven track record, profitability, or predictable revenue. Afterwards, if more capital is required, equity can be issued in a series of "rounds."

Early equity rounds are typically the purview of "venture capital," which is private equity in which there is high risk due to the newness of the idea or business. Venture capitalists assume many startups will fail, but a few may be highly profitable, so they will place bets based on high risk and high expectations for return from those businesses that do succeed. For founders, the tradeoff is loss of controlling equity stakes for the ongoing survival of the business. Venture capitalists can also bring business acumen and adequate capital to create scale (and therefore expected large returns on the investment), but often do so with expectations of strategic control of the business.

As businesses become more predictable, later rounds of equity investment may come not from the early high-risk venture capitalists but from the more conservative "mid-market" and "late-market" private equity investors looking for a steady rate of return on investment, or adequate capital to grow a thriving and successful business to a larger scale. Many private equity funds are pooled funds raised from high-net-worth individuals or businesses, and their business model is often built on putting in equity for growth or profit improvement purposes and then exiting the investment within an approximate three-to-five-year horizon. At the end of that time, the fund will often pay out its investors and sell the business to private equity investors with a longer, more conservative time horizon, or ready the business for the public markets.

Medical groups in the past did not have access to private equity, because corporate practice of medicine laws in most states precluded non-physician owners from investing in medical practices. However, the development of strategies based on long-term contractual relationships between medical practices and private equity investors in management services arrangements has allowed the entry of private equity investment into the medical practice markets.

Private equity investors often target potentially highly profitable medical specialties that can be more profitable with efficient management and scalable services. Health systems have argued that these arrangements skim off the efficient services and leave the less-profitable local healthcare services for the hospitals to manage, but without the cross-subsidization that the lucrative services often allow. The private equity-owned practices argue that their efficiently run practices are more cost-effective in mature healthcare markets than inefficient hospital-run practices.

Bond and Stock Markets: Hospital systems have access to differing types of capital depending on how they are organized. For-profit hospitals, which make up about 24% of community hospitals in the United States, pay taxes and can access capital through private or public equity markets. Some states have a much larger share of for-profit hospitals, including Nevada (54%), Texas (52%), Florida (48%), New Mexico (43%), Arizona (41%), and Louisiana (41%). About 58% of community hospitals are nonprofit, and 19% are government-owned by state or local governments. [103]

Nonprofit hospitals primarily access capital through a combination of revenue generated from patient services, investments, philanthropic donations, government grants, and by issuing tax-exempt bonds in the bond market, essentially borrowing money while benefiting from lower interest rates due to their nonprofit status.

Essentially, the difference between for-profit and nonprofit hospitals is how they access capital and what the expectations are that result from those sources of capital. For-profit entities have obligations to shareholders for an expected return on investment. Nonprofit organizations, due to their tax-exempt status, often have obligations to demonstrate community benefit. Both types of institutions provide charity care.

Over the course of the past decade, large publicly traded companies have invested directly in medical practices. The largest employer of physicians in the United States currently is Optum Health, a division of UnitedHealthcare, ranked eighth on the 2024 Fortune Global 500 list of publicly traded companies. Other publicly traded companies, such as traditional healthcare companies like Humana and CVS, also have physician practices, but nontraditional publicly traded companies such as Amazon and Walmart are also investing in medical practices.

WINNERS, LOSERS, AND THE CONSEQUENCES OF CAPITAL ACCESS

The bottom line is that sources of revenue to provide healthcare services are extraordinarily varied, and have massively complex regulatory and business payment criteria, while the business models of healthcare companies themselves are equally complex, with varying sources of capital, each with their own business expectations and time frames for return on investment. The result is that a substantial amount of healthcare complexity and inefficiency falls on the backs of front-line providers who are faced with requirements for payment, which often make up most of the chores they face in their daily professional lives.

Different individuals and institutions within the healthcare delivery system have varying levels of access to capital in its various forms. The results of the differential in access create winners and losers in terms of their ability to innovate and succeed in the complex healthcare ecosystem. Organizations with access to capital can scale and make infrastructure investments, attract and retain talent, and may be more likely to take strategic risks, provided the capital structure they are obligated to gives a return that meets their expectations. Those with limited capital access may tend to limit care innovation and are constrained by their ability to survive transitions in business models.

Understanding the financial engine behind healthcare reveals the forces that shape every workflow, every obstacle, and every moment of clinician frustration. To eliminate the chores, we must first follow the money.

CHAPTER 28

Hospitals as Airports: Rethinking Healthcare through System Design

n 1999, while in graduate school earning my master's in medical management, I read an article titled "The Hospital as Airport: A New Model for Health Care."[104] The premise has stayed with me: Hospitals could learn a great deal from the design of airports.

The author makes the point that an airport is set up in a business model where it does not own all the business processes that go on there. Rather, it serves as an integrated physical hub where multiple businesses that make up the airline industry ecosystem interact to provide services that are more than the sum of the parts: airline companies, the TSA, food vendors, ground transportation businesses, maintenance businesses, and air traffic control, to name a few.

Hospitals, in contrast, have pursued vertical integration — attempting to own and manage nearly every function in the healthcare delivery system, irrespective of their capacity to perform those subservices effectively and efficiently. As a consequence, hospitals have merged over the past 30 years to form large integrated healthcare systems where the business model has prioritized full vertical integration — owning everything from physician practices to facility maintenance and billing departments. The assumption is that scale is associated with increased efficiencies and high profitability, and that "ownership" is necessary for this scale and efficiency.

Like airports, hospitals are distinct physical spaces where highly complex processes based on aggregations of technology function to provide healthcare services. What airports recognize, however, is that these aggregated businesses should be organized around passenger service needs rather than around a single vertical ownership model. Thus, those experts at moving baggage do so, those focused on providing food do so, and those focused on landing planes do so.

In contrast, hospitals have tended to try to own physicians, employ their own maintenance services, and do their own revenue cycle management. As the costs of administrative and clinical workflows increase, with inadequate local expertise in many markets and with the advent of new forms of technology, including 24/7 remote clinical and administrative support, an "airport" model may end up being the most viable business model for the future of healthcare.

New and more sustainable business models can develop when we understand the individual chores necessary to provide services at a deep level. Focus on the end-user — the patient needing care — is step one. Step two is determining whether the way services are provided currently is actually the best way to provide them. Does everything have to be done in a clinic or hospital inpatient setting? Or, can a significant amount of healthcare be provided more efficiently and equally effectively in the home, or digitally, irrespective of location, at any time, day or night?

For services that must be provided in intensive care units or operating rooms, what types of workflows must be done by the hospital itself versus others? Does any amount of revenue cycle management actually require local resources? How much of the clinical workflow can be done remotely? Can global human resources improve local care by offering a labor market that is open 24/7, 365 days a year, rather than the typical service level now provided at hospitals, which is often substandard on weekends compared to weekdays?

Over the past few years, hospitals have begun to outsource various components of their workflow to companies that are focused entirely on that aspect, such as revenue cycle management, in ways that lead to cost reduction and efficiency not obtainable with local resources only.

The use of artificial intelligence will increase this trend as costs continue to decrease with the improvement in information infrastructure at the global management level. However, the largest gains may actually come from the improvement in clinical processes and workflows. As this occurs, much of what makes up the local hospital system ecosystem may have to be reconstrued, and the "airport" model of integrator and aggregator in a non-ownership model may be a far more efficient business model henceforth.

By understanding which processes are "core" to patient care and which are administrative chores, hospitals can begin designing service layers that are more nimble, efficient, and patient-centered. Just as airports adapted to

CHAPTER 28: Hospitals as Airports: Rethinking Healthcare through System Design | **133**

serve millions efficiently by coordinating rather than controlling, the future hospital must evolve into a care hub — integrated, patient-centered, and agile — not bound by the inefficiencies of ownership, but empowered by intelligent design.

CHAPTER 29

Global Human Capital and Pragmatic Technology

T he future of healthcare delivery lies in blending global human capital with pragmatic, human-centered technology. This shift challenges outdated assumptions that every healthcare function must be performed locally. Harvard business scholar Clay Christensen noted that the 20th-century U.S. healthcare system was built around expensive, localized care hubs because travel was expensive. So, communities required investment in expensive local technologies to supply 20th-century healthcare based on the need to aggregate expensive resources for surgeries, advanced imaging, diagnostic testing, and advanced therapeutics.[31]

Over the course of the 20th century, from the post-World War II enactment of the Hill-Burton Act that focused on remedying access to good healthcare by investing in local hospitals across the country, each community developed hubs of aggregated healthcare resources that, for better or worse, have become the largest employers in nearly every community in the country.

This model made a lot of sense in 1945, but not so much anymore. There is often a lack of access to adequate healthcare workers, and it is expensive for many of these jobs to be done locally in every community. It creates duplication, inefficiency, and prohibits appropriate scaling. Christensen pointed out that travel is now far less expensive, yet we will have a business model built on having a redundancy of resources in local markets, where quality might improve and costs decrease with resources distributed more rationally based on centers of excellence for many services.

Today, real-time video conferencing, broadband internet, and AI-enabled tools enable us to redesign clinical and administrative services around global capabilities. Teleradiology enables sub-specialized image interpretation from anywhere in the world, improving accuracy and turnaround times. Robotic surgery offers the potential for complex procedures to be performed remotely. At a more routine level, day-to-day administrative and clinical support — such as real-time medical scribing — can be provided by trained professionals worldwide, delivering high-quality support 24/7.

My company can provide real-time scribing to physicians around the world 24/7 because we have a highly trained clinical workforce fluent in English and medically trained in every time zone. A physician practicing in a rural setting in the Midwest might have a very different experience if their only resource is local. Additionally, the deep evaluation of what tasks must be done locally versus those that traditionally have been done locally can redesign work such that the tasks performed in the local setting are more patient-focused and meaningful.

To achieve this transformation, we must answer three key questions:

- **What tasks must be done locally?**
- **What tasks can be done remotely?**
- **What tasks require human input and which can be automated?**

These questions must be guided by a commitment to pragmatic technology — tools that serve the people doing the work rather than humans serving the tool. There is a need to avoid the "gee whiz" factor of technology for technology's sake and instead focus on what makes the work of human beings easier within the constraints of human-centered design.

Current electronic health record design often violates this principle, putting my skills as a highly trained physician and putting them into a data entry workflow. At least 70% of what the electronic health record I use in my clinical practice demands for clinical documentation does not require my medical degree, nor should it be done by me. In the near future, there should be a structure where human-centered technology does what technology does best, and the human workforce is divided into the global workforce that can do work from anywhere, the local workforce that is required in the immediate care setting, and the professionals performing work that is at the top of their license rather than, as it often feels in my clinic, at the bottom.

A thoughtfully integrated global workforce and pragmatic, human-centered technology enable healthcare to be redesigned from the ground up. If properly structured, this model can deliver higher-quality care at lower cost, with greater consistency. But design matters: Systems must preserve safety and trust, with appropriate "humans in the loop." Sometimes that human needs to be an expert. Other times, what's needed is not expertise at all, but empathy, presence, and the capacity to truly listen.

CHAPTER 30

Rethinking the Healthcare Team: Beyond the Lone Physician

Over the past 20 years, the archetype of the lone, heroic physician has given way to the reality of team-based care. The demands of modern medicine — exponentially growing knowledge, specialized technologies, and complex patient needs — have made solo practice both unrealistic and inefficient.

In response, care delivery has shifted toward integrated teams, where professionals work at the top of their license and training to collectively meet patient needs. Team-based care is not only preferable, but also essential. The transformation has been a matter of necessity, as the knowledge upon which medical care is based has grown beyond the capabilities of an individual physician to acquire, with technologies that are highly sophisticated requiring highly specialized training and skills, and complex needs of patients that extend beyond the individual acute transaction to aspects of communication, longitudinal care, and comprehensive medication management. Teams of people are far more capable of providing complex care than individual physicians are.

While the image of a physician on horseback making house calls remains a romanticized part of our cultural memory, today's medical challenges — from genomic medicine to longitudinal chronic disease management — require coordination, not individual heroics.

As healthcare became more technologically advanced, hospitals became the first places for team-based care. The operating room was the earliest example of effective team-based care. Surgeons, anesthesiologists, nurses, and technologists demonstrated how coordinated efforts could achieve results that no one professional could accomplish alone. From this environment came early quality standards, including those later institutionalized by The Joint Commission. Later on, it was anesthesiologists in the operating room setting who first advanced six sigma level performance in certain aspects of healthcare related to surgical outcomes.

Teams are focused on working together such that everyone has a unique role that allows for more efficient and effective delivery of services. Healthcare today is less a one-man band and more a symphony. Each professional plays a distinct role, coordinated toward a common goal: better outcomes, reduced errors, and sustainable workloads. And within the context of the chores of healthcare, working everyone at the top of their license actually reduces the chores an individual has, because chores are distributed, and the chores of one person may be the core function of someone else on the team. Work that feels like a chore to one clinician may be the core competency — and even the passion — of another. When tasks are distributed wisely, everyone operates closer to their purpose.

It is essential to consider teams in a broad context. With technology and global human capital, a team can be distributed across the globe. Key design questions for future-ready care teams include:

- Does this task require a physician — or could it be better handled by a nurse, pharmacist, care coordinator, or scribe?
- Does it need to occur in a clinic — or could it be done virtually, asynchronously, or in the home?
- Does it require a human — or could automation safely handle it?

A recent framing of the problem of dysfunctional clinical work environments has highlighted the concept of attention and how health systems design can impact patient care quality and medical errors by "paying attention to attention." Kissler and colleagues emphasized that an "ecology of attention" can serve as a useful guiding framework with which to understand the needs of clinicians and the impact of health systems design on patient care:

> "A clinician's typical workday involves careful decision making, technical expertise, and often, moments of deep human connection. All of this work can be meaningful and satisfying and, to be done well, requires a clinician's full attention. However, care environments do not always facilitate a state of attention, leading to harm for both patients (medical errors) and clinicians (burnout). Patient complexity continues to increase, as measured by various characteristics including multimorbidity, polypharmacy, and risk for readmission, while the complexity of the systems and tasks required of the clinician navigating care systems is also increasing. Cognitive failures and attentional lapses contribute to medical errors and, sometimes the well-intentioned efforts to avoid them create environments that are less amenable to the interpersonal and individualized work of care. Reorganizing care

around these questions allows each team member to contribute where they add the most value, reducing inefficiency and clinician burnout."[105]

Their framework provides an additional window into how human-centered design could be utilized to affect the "ecology of clinician attention" such that key measurable factors that influence the ability of clinicians to maintain presence and focus can be analyzed. Barriers to attention in the salient work environment include workload and alarms and alerts, inappropriate triage, interruptions and distractions, and unnecessary non-clinical tasks. These attention disruptors can be reengineered around pragmatic technology and a global human workforce to provide a safer and more sustainable work environment for clinicians and their staffs.

CHAPTER 31

Patients vs. Consumers

For those of us trained in medicine, the shift toward describing the people we care for as "consumers" rather than "patients" represents a fundamental change — not just in language, but in philosophy — and it has not always been easy to accept. The word *patient* derives from the concept of someone who is "acted upon," from the Latin word *"patiens,"* meaning *"to suffer."* From this perspective, the relationship between the physician and their patient is developed within the context of the professional relationship and its associated ethical boundaries.

Consumers, on the other hand, are defined as those who utilize economic goods. Much has been written over the past decade to emphasize that we should be treating our patients more as consumers. Consumers typically have a choice and make economic decisions in their own self-interest, focused on the perceived value of a consumed good relative to the price they are willing to pay for it. The idea that someone is a consumer of healthcare services implies they may become more involved in their own healthcare needs, and services may be better designed around price, convenience, outcome, and unmet needs.

These distinctions are not entirely helpful when it comes to aspects of the human condition that occur as a result of significant medical illness. It may be easy for someone with relatively minor medical needs, such as treatment for a simple urinary tract infection, to view their care within the context of a consumer mindset. They may prioritize fast, conveniently accessible care, expect an accurate diagnosis, and be provided with the right medication. But the diagnosis of cancer, end-stage renal disease, or a serious neurodegenerative condition such as multiple sclerosis presents a different scenario. Where suffering is profound and clinical expertise essential, the traditional patient role — and the need for trust in the clinician — becomes paramount.

Despite the tensions, some argue that healthcare consumerism is a necessary driver of patient-centered care.[106] Provider centrism assumes that physicians know "what's best" for patients, whereas healthcare consumerism focuses on what the consumer demands from the providers. Unfortunately, an asymmetry of information remains inherent in the expertise of trained medical professionals and patients suffering from conditions that they do not control and often cannot affect without the help of the healthcare provider.

The consumer of healthcare typically is not the one paying for the service, which further complicates the drive for choice and value. The advent of artificial intelligence will drive changes in the natural asymmetry of information between physicians and patients, but it will not eliminate it. Therefore, the mindful design of the practice of the future will consider the change in access to information.

Those who disagree with the position that patient-centrism and consumerism are one and the same typically disagree with its market focus:

> "Today's consumer-drive health care has become associated with neoliberal efforts to emphasize market factors in health reform and de-emphasize government regulation and financing. In our view, a narrow focus on consumerism is conceptually confusing and potentially harmful. The consumer metaphor wrongly assumes that healthcare is a market in the usual understanding of that term, that the high cost of US health care is a function of excessive consumer demand, and that price transparency and competition can deliver on the promise of reducing costs or ensuring quality. Furthermore, a consumer metaphor places disproportionate burdens on patients to reduce health care costs, and it could erode professional obligations to provide appropriate and effective care."[107]

> "When patients are healthy, convenience is prioritized. When a patient is chronically ill or hospitalized, coordination steps to the forefront. When a patient is actually ill or injured, access is most important.[108]

> "Here's my question: How did it become normal, or for that matter even acceptable to refer to medical patients as 'consumers'? The relationship between patient and doctor used to be considered something special, almost sacred. Now, politicians and supposed reformers talk about the act of receiving care as if it were no different from a commercial transaction, like buying a car, and their only complaint is that it isn't commercial enough. What has gone wrong with us?"[109]

The focus on consumerism presumes that consumers have decision-making power. However, patients who are suffering are vulnerable and must put their lives in the hands of medical professionals who have a responsibility to do what is best for the patient. Their care is often paid for by a third party.

Within the context of core versus chore, we can distinguish the core mission of a medical provider as being the medical care and treatment of the patient, and perhaps the core mission of a medical business as providing the best value for a consumer of medical services. By refusing the false dichotomy of the distinction, a system can be designed around the quadruple aim of best care for the patient at the right place at the right time — something that is compatible with both points of view.

Understanding when a person is best served as a vulnerable patient versus as an empowered consumer is essential. Designing with this dual perspective enables us to streamline administrative chores while strengthening trust and agency. Rather than choosing between two incompatible identities, we might accept that individuals move fluidly between roles. A person may be a consumer when comparing health plans, a patient when receiving a serious diagnosis, and a caregiver when helping a family member navigate complex care. A well-designed system accommodates these shifts with empathy, flexibility, and clarity.

CHAPTER 32

Precision Medicine Is Patient-Centered

P recision medicine is, at its core, the clinical embodiment of patient-centered care. As Claude Bernard noted in 1865, "*A physician is by no means physician to living beings in general, not even physician to the human race, but rather, physician to a human individual in certain morbid conditions peculiar to himself and forming what is called his idiosyncrasy.*"[110] Precision medicine is a medical model that separates people into different groups, with medical decisions, practices, interventions and/or products being tailored to the individual patients based on their predicted response or risk of disease.[111] As we redesign healthcare to eliminate unnecessary chores, it is crucial that we understand the profound changes in workflow processes that precision medicine may have on the industry.

In 2011, as a founding member of the Oliver Wyman Healthcare Innovation Center, I worked with colleagues to forecast three successive waves of healthcare transformation:

- **Wave One (2011–2016):** A shift from volume to value, refocusing healthcare on patient-centered care and reimbursement tied to outcomes.
- **Wave Two (2014–2020):** Consumer engagement and digital tools to empower individuals in their own health decisions.
- **Wave Three (2018–2025):** The science of prevention — using genomic and data-driven insights to create precision medicine tailored to the individual.

In our vision of wave three, the convergence of big data aligning insights from the exposome with genome, proteome, and microbiome, integrating data in the electronic health record and the patient's personal health record, indicating pharmacogenomic interactions to target personalized therapies would create a new paradigm that focused not on the "socialized" medicine of averages and clinical trials, but a new type of medical built on a "n" of one. That is, the precise treatment a single individual might best respond to is determined and implemented rather than relying on clinical trials based on large populations of patients with various genetic profiles and responses to treatment.

It is quite true that our idealized view of the three waves has yet to be fulfilled; however, it is equally true that there has been movement on value-based care, consumer engagement, and precision medicine. Almost all of Medicare will be paid in some form of value contract by 2030. Consumer engagement has accelerated with the use of healthcare apps, and health systems are starting to build out digital front doors on top of traditional ways of delivering care. The confluence of whole genome sequencing for $100 or less and AI-driven forms of data integration and analysis will exponentially accelerate the potential of precision medicine.

However, headwinds threaten the third wave. Despite technological advances, clinicians and systems are unprepared. While the vast majority of physicians acknowledge that genomics influences treatment, only a tiny minority feel adequately trained to use it in clinical practice. This knowledge gap, coupled with the shortage of clinical geneticists and genetic counselors, presents a critical barrier.

Evidence-based practice guidelines have not been developed for most genetic testing. In an American Medical Association survey of more than 10,000 physicians, 98% indicated they are aware that patient genomics influences response to drug therapy, but only 10% believe they are adequately informed and comfortable with using genetic information to guide treatment in clinical practice. There are currently more than 75,000 individual genetic testing products on the United States market, with 10 new tests entering the market every day, yet there are currently fewer than 1,000 practicing clinical geneticists in the United States and only 2,000 genetic counselors.[112]

Precision medicine disrupts the traditional economics of healthcare. The blockbuster drug model, based on large populations and average outcomes, struggles in a world of individualized care. Diagnostic tools that narrow treatment populations may reduce market size for some therapies while making others newly viable.

The traditional business model of the pharmaceutical industry has been built on blockbuster drugs that are approved based on research evaluating average patient efficacy and safety data. Diagnostic tests, biomarkers, and targeted treatments are altering traditional research methods and economic funding models on which the industry is based. Molecular diagnostics can determine which patients may benefit or be harmed by a drug, thereby narrowing the indications and market for some therapies while permitting some medications previously deemed too unsafe to be reintroduced with companion diagnostics.

The current fee-for-service payment system is poorly adapted for precision medicine. Although more than 75,000 genetic tests are available, there are only 500 separate Current Procedural Terminology (CPT) codes under which they are billed. Actuarial science, predictive risk, and economic models are not well-designed to integrate with the science of individuality ("n of one") inherent in personalized medicine.

Studies linking companion diagnostics to improved health outcomes are often unavailable or poorly understood by the payer community. Typically, there is no payment for diagnostics that stratify the population. The unit costs of individual tests do not necessarily align with their potentially outsized impact on the total cost of care in current actuarial models.

The policy makers at the federal level are equally ill-prepared for precision medicine. Genetic data has implications not only for individual patients but also for their family members. Policy balancing the need for data-sharing to advance medical knowledge with privacy issues has not been adequately implemented. Regulatory bodies must ensure that frameworks are in place to safeguard patients while guaranteeing that scientific progress is not hampered.

Despite the hurdles, the potential of precision medicine remains transformational. Its care model is often defined by the "Four Ps": Predictive, Preventive, Personalized, and Participatory. Its benefits include:

- Shifting care from reaction to prevention.
- Predicting disease susceptibility.
- Improving early detection.
- Preempting progression.
- Tailoring prevention and treatment strategies.
- Avoiding harmful side effects.
- Reducing drug development time and cost.
- Eliminating trial-and-error inefficiencies.

Rather than a "one drug/procedure/treatment fits all" approach, diagnostic testing, imaging analysis, molecular and cellular analysis, and analytics can be employed to tailor medical treatment to the individual characteristics of each patient. Disease risk assessment can be built into prevention and treatment initiatives for patients before a disease even manifests, and artificial intelligence is being used to draw inferences from big data sources to improve the quality of patient care, enable cost-effectiveness, and reduce readmission and mortality rates.

Yet precision medicine will not escape the burdens of the current system. It will create new chores — from unfiltered test recommendations in EHRs to delays in specialist referrals. In my own practice, a recent EHR upgrade began flagging genetic counseling needs for Lynch syndrome based on opaque logic, sending me down rabbit holes for justification and hitting a wall of limited referral capacity. Precision medicine's promise will only be fulfilled if we proactively design systems that eliminate these new chores, not add to them.

CHAPTER 33

Population Health and the Rubik's Cube: A Framework for Human-Centered Redesign

Healthcare delivery is undeniably complex — but it is also solvable. The focus of this book is to distinguish between the *chores* that burden the system and the *core* mission of delivering patient care. By eliminating unnecessary tasks, enabling every team member to work at the top of their training and licensure, and using human-centered design, we can redesign workflows to improve satisfaction and reduce burnout.

Population health management provides a valuable lens through which to apply these redesign principles. In the context of population health, understanding the multiple dimensions and how they work together is a crucial way of thinking through these improvements.

In a dream — much like August Kekulé's vision of a snake biting its tail that led to his discovery of benzene's ring structure — I imagined a Rubik's Cube as a metaphor for the dimensions of population health. Each side of the cube represented one aspect of the healthcare system, with eight subdivisions per face. When mixed up, the cube captured the tangled, chaotic nature of healthcare delivery. But like the actual Rubik's Cube, if we understand its structure, we can solve it — systematically, creatively, and with clarity. Here is what I imagine should be on the six faces if population health:

Face 1: Population Segments

1. Healthy
2. Healthy with Risk Factors
3. Healthy with Acute Limited Conditions
4. Early-Stage Chronic Disease
5. Complex Conditions
6. Poly-Chronic Conditions
7. Late-Stage Conditions
8. End-of-Life

Face 2: Types of Medical Conditions

1. Independent Conditions
2. Prevalence-Sensitive Conditions
3. Episodic Conditions
4. Progressive Conditions
5. Degenerative Conditions
6. Systemic Conditions
7. Heritable Conditions
8. Socially Determined Conditions

Face 3: Episodes of Care

1. Preventative Services
2. Routine Care
3. Minor Episodic Care
4. Major Episodic Care
5. Catastrophic Care
6. Long-Term Care
7. Home Care
8. Palliative Care

Face 4: Managed Care Components

1. Benefits Design
2. Pre-Authorization
3. Co-Pays
4. Deductibles
5. Wellness Programs
6. Tiered Formularies
7. Co-Insurance
8. HMOs / PPOs / Narrow Networks

Face 5: Payment Models

1. Fee-for-Service
2. Care Coordination Payments
3. Pay-for-Performance
4. Episode Bundles
5. Chronic Condition Bundles
6. Shared Savings
7. Shared Risk
8. Full Capitation

Face 6: Care Delivery Models

1. Primary Care / Patient-Centered Medical Home (PCMH)
2. Specialty Condition-Based Medical Homes
3. Telehealth
4. Community / Public Health
5. Integrated Delivery Systems
6. Accountable Care Organizations (ACOs)
7. Self-Care / Social Networks
8. Faith-Based Models

Like the Rubik's Cube, healthcare's many components are often jumbled: population needs, payment models, care delivery systems, benefits design, and more. Solving the puzzle means understanding how these faces interconnect. If we can structure our thinking around the six domains — population segment, medical condition, episode of care, managed care, payment policy, and care model — we can develop highly personalized, scalable systems of care. This framework transforms chaos into solvable complexity and reaffirms that healthcare — when thoughtfully designed around human needs — is not only fixable, but improvable.

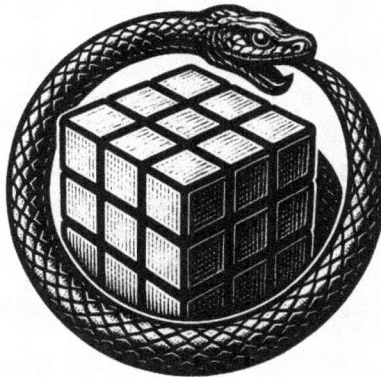

CHAPTER 34

Fixing Our Broken Healthcare System by Understanding Non-Western Culture's Approaches to Health and Well-Being

"To think better, to think like the best humans, we are probably going to have to learn again to judge a person's intelligence, not by the ability to recite facts, but by the good order or harmoniousness of his or her surroundings."[113]

In 2010, I was introduced to a non-Western conception of health and well-being as expressed by the Eastern band of Cherokees in western North Carolina, or as they were traditionally called, the Kituwah people. Their standard greeting is *"Siyo! Tohi-tsu*?", or "Hello, are you well?" This is not a Cherokee equivalent of the English, "Hello, how are you?" Rather, it embodies the Cherokee view of the workings of the cosmos and the position of the individual in relationship to the rest of the world.

Tohi is the Cherokee word for wellness, "an ideal state of being, peace." The word is meant to emphasize that you are in good health when your body and mind are at peace. Within this context, health is more than the absence of disease; it includes a fully confident sense of a smooth life, peaceful existence, unhurried pace, and easy flow of time. Tohi means "not tense, not rushed, not agitated, your body's not working hard, and everything's flowing smoothly." The fluidity and balance of tohi can be disrupted through illness, aggravation, and simply being out of sorts or *nohsana*.

The Cherokee word for a disease of the body is *ahyugi*, which means an angry or resentful entity that comes to visit. A person who has a chronic illness is *uwehi,* "illness that lives in the body." "*Agwohiyu nohasana yige-sesdi*" means "I think that it will not turn out well in the future." "*Kilogohusdi nagwvneha*" means "someone is making my state of being a certain way," reflecting the notion that one's normal state of being is being manipulated and altered by another person.

These terms all demonstrate a Cherokee world in which a central feature is that it should be fluid, peaceful, and easy like water flowing. The proper state of the Cherokee individual is centered, balanced, and neutral. When an individual does something to deviate from the state of tohi, illness or other consequences befall them. Only by engaging in healing that restores the world and the individual to the appropriate state can things be made right again.[114]

As modern medicine catches up with the Cherokee perspective that health is a matter of balance, and that stress, poverty, and trauma can make you sick, the traditional holistic perspective of the Cherokee medicine man is to figure out how to bring back balance to restore health. They perceive social and medical manifestations of unbalanced change to be a "soul wound," a term implying deep "trauma seen, felt, and heard is transformed deep with the psyche and erupts into forms of abusive, anxious, and depressive behaviors resulting from generations of exploitation, assimilation and marginalization."[114]

To achieve Tohi, the Cherokee believe that one must understand how things in the world work or function in the right way, or *duyuk'dv'i.* Cherokee spiritual healer Tom Belt describes the importance of *duyuk'dv'i,* in achieving *Tohi.* "The Kituwah way is to use language to heal, and it reflects living a life on the right path, *duyuk'dv'i,* the right way, the right path." To be out of *Tohi* is to be out of balance.[114]

From a human-centered design perspective, the Cherokee concept of *Tohi* exemplifies a design approach rooted in empathy, balance, and contextual understanding. Rather than isolating symptoms or problems from their environments — as Western medicine often does — Cherokee healing systems view wellness as a dynamic state influenced by social, emotional, and spiritual forces. This systems-aware, empathic model echoes the principles of design thinking: start with empathy, define the problem in context, ideate holistic solutions, and prototype for a better, more balanced human experience.

Many other global perspectives could help bridge design thinking for healthcare professionals:

Ubuntu (Southern Africa)

In many African cultures, especially among the Zulu and Xhosa, the concept of *Ubuntu* — "I am because we are" — guides well-being. Health is seen as embedded in the strength of community relationships. Disconnection from one's social group is considered a source of emotional and even physical illness. *Ubuntu*, like tohi, highlights balance and relational harmony as essential for healing.

Ayurveda (India)

In traditional Indian Ayurvedic medicine, health is achieved when the three doshas (*vata, pitta, kapha*) are in balance. These are energetic forces that represent the body, mind, and lifestyle. Illness is a manifestation of imbalance — just as burnout in Western physicians may reflect disconnection from the "right path." Design thinking rooted in Ayurvedic insight would focus on personalized, context-specific solutions that restore equilibrium.

Māori Hauora (New Zealand)

The Māori model of *hauora* defines health as a balance across four pillars: physical, mental/emotional, family/social, and spiritual well-being. This quadrilateral model offers a literal design frame for visualizing health as a system rather than a list of symptoms. When any pillar is unstable, the whole structure falters—mirroring the "soul wound" and imbalance you describe.

What does this all have to do with "core versus chore"? As physicians, our core mission is to heal people, but we are currently confronted with an unbalanced profession that has become uprooted from our core mission. Our chores are like a disease. We are unbalanced, uprooted, and not living right. As a result, we have experienced a "soul wound," which explains our burnout and professional despair.

To return to a state of *Tohi*, we certainly need to determine how to return to the right path, how to live as physicians in the right way. In my mind, the term "moral injury," which has become the dominant paradigm in Western medicine, is a close cousin to the Cherokee "soul wound." We must turn to that now to identify Western ways of applying the right way of living to return our profession to health.

While Western medicine excels at isolating and treating disease, it often fails to see the patient — or the physician — as part of an interconnected system of balance, purpose, and relationship. By learning from Indigenous and non-Western perspectives, and incorporating these into our design methodologies, we can begin to reimagine health not just as survival, but as harmony. Not just the absence of illness, but the presence of meaning.

CHAPTER 35

Design for Wellville: A Human-Centered Approach Beyond the Social Determinants of Health

A round 2012, I met Esther Dyson through the Oliver Wyman Health Innovation Leadership Alliance. An early tech investor, a prolific writer, a backup astronaut for the International Space Station, and — most relevant here — the founder of Wellville, Esther has spent the last decade working to improve equitable well-being in five diverse U.S. communities.

Wellville wasn't just another social determinants of health (SDoH) program. It was a living experiment in community-centered, design-driven health creation. Rather than merely identifying disparities, it asked three deceptively simple questions:

- What future do we want?
- What's holding us back?
- What will it take to get there?

Wellville was a 10-year national nonprofit project focused on serving as a catalyst for five communities in the United States as they worked to improve their health and well-being through resident-centered, multi-stakeholder collaboration. The five Wellville communities, Clatsop County, Oregon, Lake County, California, Muskego, Michigan, North Hartford, Connecticut, and Spartanburg, South Carolina, each engaged with the Wellville nonprofit to reimagine how they might support long, healthy lives for everyone.

Each community developed its own processes to answer three questions:[115]

- **Spartanburg** launched the SIREN initiative to shift power toward Black residents affected by past urban renewal. The Spartanburg Initiative for

Racial Equity Now (SIREN) advocated for a shift in how community development decisions are made, proposing a more central role for residents of the primarily Black neighborhoods that have been decimated by urban renewal.

- **Clatsop County** worked to amplify Hispanic voices in decision-making. Clatsop County team members strategized on ways to elevate the priorities of the Hispanic population.
- **North Hartford** built civic momentum around ending food deserts. North Harford residents and organization leaders shared their stories of self, stories of us now, deepening their relationships and resolving to bring a grocery store to an area of the city that has been deemed a food desert and a food swamp.
- **Muskegon** invested in nurturing the next generation of health equity leaders. These changemakers empowered the new leaders to pursue the changes they want to see.
- **Lake County** reached out to Native American communities to co-create a shared plan for well-being. The Lake County team mapped out a community engagement process, including more international outreach to Native Americans, to create a shared plan for countywide health improvement.

What ties these stories together is not a shared playbook, but a shared design thinking mindset:

- They empathized with residents.
- They defined their own challenges.
- They ideated community-driven solutions.
- They prototyped new programs.
- They tested and iterated based on what actually mattered.

This is design thinking, not as a workshop tool, but as a philosophy of collaborative, place-based transformation. In Wellville, community health was not a product to be delivered; it was a system to be co-created.

These approaches do not sound like classical engineering for problem-solving, but their strategic approach is built on listening empathetically and generatively, revealing ground truths about the causes of harm and health, imagining new futures, and moving forward together by learning, adjusting through messes, breakdowns, and potential opportunities that emerge along the way. his approach has led to a number of community-led actions with long-term shared investments and shared benefits in early childhood education, paths out of homelessness, diabetes prevention, food access, and equity and inclusion.

This type of broad reimagining of how to affect health outcomes gets at much of what is missing from the current healthcare solutions thought process and likely provides its antidote. In the United States, average life expectancy varies across different segments of the population. The richest American men live 15 years longer than the poorest men, while the richest American women live 10 years longer than the poorest women. These gaps between rich and poor are growing rapidly over time.[116]

Life expectancy in the United States by ethnicity is even more varied, with Asian Americans living on average 84.5 years, white Americans 77.5, Hispanic Americans 80, Black Americans 72.8, and American Indians and Alaska Natives 67.9 years. Gender data indicate women live on average 81.1 years and men 75.8.

Large decreases in life expectancy between 2019 and 2021 disproportionately impacted historically disadvantaged groups with marked deaths among people of color.

The factors driving disparities in life expectancy are complex and multifactorial and include differences in health insurance coverage and access to care, social and economic factors, and health behaviors that are rooted in structural and systemic racism and discrimination (see Table 6).[117]

TABLE 6. Health Disparities Are Driven by Economic and Social Disparities

Economic Stability	Neighborhood and Physical Environment	Education	Food	Community, Safety, and Social Context	Healthcare System	Discrimination
Employment	Housing	Literacy	Food security	Social integration	Health coverage	Ethnic
Income	Transportation	Language	Access to healthy options	Support systems	Provider & pharmacy availability	Gender
Expenses	Parks	Early childhood education		Community engagement	Access to linguistically and culturally appropriate & respectful care	Racial
Debt	Playgrounds	Vocational training		Stress		
Medical bills	Walkability	Higher education		Exposure to violence/trauma		
Support	Zip code/ geography			Policing/justice policy	Quality of care	
	Urban vs Rural					

Taking control of the social determinants of health as part of the chores to be addressed in new ways will likely lower the administrative burden and total cost of care, while also improving outcomes. Much of the moral injury that physicians experience can be attributed to the frustration and disappointment of not being able to positively affect the health of more patients due to factors outside the control of office workflow. Most healthcare systems treat social needs as adjunct chores — check-the-box items for screening or referral. But Wellville inverted this logic, asking: "What if addressing food access, safe housing, and social cohesion were part of our core design for health creation?"

When communities are built around well-being, the burden on individual clinicians decreases. The chore of care coordination becomes shared across sectors, no longer the sole responsibility of primary care teams. This is where design meets equity — and reduces burnout at the root. When physicians are unable to meaningfully affect the health of patients whose lives are shaped by poverty, trauma, or housing insecurity, the result is moral injury. The current healthcare system turns those failures into daily chores: referral checklists, documentation burdens, and frustrated follow-ups.

However, if we design for well-being rather than disease management, and if we build communities that nurture health rather than just treat illness, we lighten the load for everyone. Wellness is not a task; it is a design challenge. And it is one that demands we expand our view of the care team to include housing advocates, food system planners, educators, employers, and — above all — patients as partners.

CHAPTER 36

Whole Person Care Matters in the Total Cost of Care

The U.S. healthcare system is widely acknowledged to be too expensive, overly complex, and prone to variability, while underdelivering on such key outcomes as life expectancy and quality of care. To reform this system effectively, we must understand the core drivers of healthcare costs and address them with a systems lens.

One major driver is demographics. One in six Americans is over the age of 65, representing nearly 20% of the population. In 2020, that translated to 56 million people. By 2030, it will be 73 million. And by 2060, more than 95 million Americans will be 65 or older — nearly one in four. Aging correlates strongly with the increased prevalence of chronic conditions. Currently, 90% of annual U.S. healthcare expenditures go toward people with chronic and mental health conditions. Three out of every four healthcare dollars are spent directly on the treatment of chronic diseases, with an additional 15% spent managing acute illnesses in patients with chronic comorbidities — who often have longer, more complicated, and costlier treatment courses.[118]

A second critical driver of costs is chronic disease itself — not just in prevalence, but in how poorly our fragmented system manages it. We lack infrastructure for longitudinal, coordinated care that meets the needs of patients holistically. This isn't just a clinical issue. It's a cost issue. Poor chronic care coordination is directly tied to avoidable hospitalizations, duplication of services, medication errors, and emergency department overutilization.

The third and perhaps most addressable cost driver is the waste baked into the structure of the system itself. According to estimates from the National Academy of Medicine and others, total waste accounts for between 25% to 30% of total U.S. healthcare spending. Let's break that down:[119]

- **Administrative complexity**: $266 billion annually due to a tangled web of payer rules, redundant documentation, regulatory variation, and security overhead.

- **Failure of care coordination**: $78 billion lost through preventable admissions, readmissions, and fragmented transitions of care.
- **Failure of care delivery**: $166 billion wasted through inefficiencies, hospital-acquired conditions, unnecessary variation, and lack of prevention.
- **Overtreatment and low-value care**: $101 billion in procedures, drugs, tests, and interventions that offer little or no benefit — or worse, cause harm.
- **Pricing failure**: $241 billion in distortions across drug, lab, and ambulatory pricing structures—often exacerbated by opaque intermediaries.
- **Fraud and abuse**: $30 billion. Though small compared to other categories, it attracts outsized political attention and distracts them from structural inefficiencies.

Every dollar wasted is a dollar diverted from meaningful care, from innovation, and from the core mission of healthcare.

This is why whole-person care — which prioritizes physical, behavioral, social, and environmental determinants of health — is so important. When care is siloed, reactive, and incomplete, costs rise and outcomes suffer. When care is connected, proactive, and holistic, people get better faster, and often at lower cost.

But here's the key insight: You cannot deliver whole-person care in a system that drowns clinicians and care teams in chores. The very waste categories listed above — administrative complexity, care coordination failure, pricing failure — are made worse by workflows that misallocate human time and attention. When physicians are overloaded with data entry, prior authorizations, inbox management, and EHR inefficiencies, their ability to coordinate, prevent, and personalize care is severely diminished.

Reducing the chore burden isn't just a matter of clinician well-being, although that matters. It's a strategic imperative. By redesigning care delivery with human-centered, team-based workflows, we can:

- Reclaim time for diagnosis, planning, and shared decision-making.
- Deploy technology to automate or delegate non-core tasks.
- Improve continuity and coordination across settings.
- Enhance cost-effectiveness at every level of the system.

When we talk about stabilizing or reducing the total cost of care, it is not an abstraction. It's a design problem. And chore elimination is a systems solution — one that touches the individual experience, organizational performance, and national sustainability of healthcare.

CHAPTER 37

How Medical Needs Are Evolving Faster Than the System Can Keep Up

"The patient is no mere collection of symptoms, signs, disordered functions, damaged organs, and disturbed emotion. He is human, fearful, and hopeful, seeking relief, help, and reassurance."[120]

I n 1900, the average life expectancy in the United States was 47 years. The death rate per 100,000 people was 1,719, and the leading causes of death were pneumonia, influenza, tuberculosis, diarrhea, and gastrointestinal diseases. Of note, these causes are all infectious diseases, for which care models were built to address acute clinical care needs.

Fifty years later, with improved public health measures in place and the advent of antibiotics for many bacterial diseases, life expectancy had risen to 68 years, with the death rate per 100,000 decreased to 963. The leading causes of death had shifted to chronic diseases like heart disease and cancer, with clinical needs modeled to take care of both acute problems and newer treatments for chronic diseases beginning to emerge.

By the time another 50 years had rolled by, life expectancy had increased in the United States to 77 years. The death rate per 100,000 in 2000 was 865, and heart disease, cancer, and cerebrovascular disease greatly outpaced acute illnesses in terms of clinical need. Heart attacks no longer routinely killed, and the diagnosis of cancer was no longer a rapid death sentence. Rather, many people were expected to live years with the diagnosis of heart disease or cancer, and much of the health system began to shift to chronic disease management and early efforts at prevention. [121]

With the tools of precision medicine, we may be able to forgo many of these chronic diseases altogether by the year 2050, but such efforts will require new tools focused on patient engagement and longitudinal care not delivered in acute or ambulatory settings. For healthcare providers, the chores of the future will evolve with the shift from chronic disease management to prevention.

The focus in the past few years on population health has been about risk-stratifying patients and developing models of care integrated with value-based payment models. The most successful population health managers have developed highly tailored care models for particular segments of the population, including those with severe behavioral illness, chronic illnesses with complex social needs, end-of-life, and those with complex and/or poly-chronic illnesses. Less focus has been placed on meeting the needs of the generally healthy or those with early or at-risk chronic conditions, and the demise of robust primary care in the United States has certainly worsened all aspects of efficient and effective care for everyone.

A recent focus of the Institute of Medicine is the improvement of the diagnostic process. The institute's goals for improving diagnosis and reducing diagnostic error emphasize the need to establish work systems and culture that support the diagnostic process and improvements in diagnostic performance, as well as a payment and care delivery environment that supports the diagnostic process.[122] The Institute of Medicine Goals for improving diagnosis and reducing diagnostic error are:

- Facilitate more effective teamwork in the diagnostic process among healthcare professionals, patients, and their families.
- Enhance healthcare professional education and training in the diagnostic process.
- Ensure that health information technologies support patients and healthcare professionals in the diagnostic process.
- Develop and deploy approaches to identify, learn from, and reduce diagnostic errors and near misses in clinical practice.
- Establish a work system and culture that supports the diagnostic process and improvements in diagnostic performance.
- Develop a reporting environment and medical liability system that facilitates improved diagnosis by learning from diagnostic errors and near misses.
- Design a payment and care delivery environment that supports the diagnostic process.
- Provide dedicated funding for research on the diagnostic process and diagnostic errors.

Much of today's healthcare improvement strategy relies on Gaussian-based statistical modeling — averages and thresholds suited to 20th-century science, but inadequate for the variability and individualization required today. Quality assurance uses an approach of creating a threshold, where action is taken below a certain point of measure, defined as "worse quality." Quality improvement methods are also built on Gaussian curves, but actions are taken on all occurrences to improve the "system" (see Figure 5.)

Likewise, the assumptions underlying healthcare payment systems have been modeled on 20th-century methodology. Actuarial risk projections are based on population averages, with trends in spending setting insurance prices. The capabilities inherent in 21st-century technology will substantially disrupt the healthcare ecosystems built on these older analytic methods.

New forms of information, including contracting expertise that incorporates alignment of incentives across contracts, effective patient segmentation and interventions, engaging and activating patients and health non-patients, functional IT systems that include analytics and workflow tools, incentives aligned with transparent clinical and financial performance metrics, high-performing provider networks, physician leadership capabilities, strategic selection of partners and community organizations, and systems of care designed around the patient versus ongoing office transformation comprise critical success factors that will be integrated in alternative payment models.

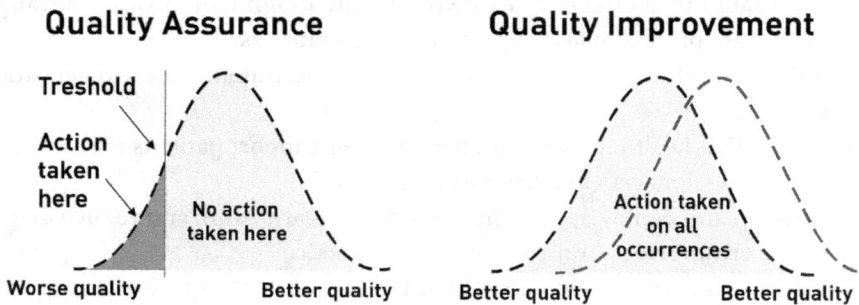

Figure 5. Typical 20th-Century Quality Methods Based on 19th-Century Mathematics.

The methods we are using to measure quality are based upon 20th-century scientific approaches and 19th-century mathematics.

The capabilities inherent in 21st-century information technology will substantially disrupt the healthcare ecosystems built on these older analytic methods. This disruption is partially the result of its scope and complexity.

In 2013, Michael Legg and the Royal College of Pathologists of Australasia presented a framework in which they argued that the application of informatics and its associated technology is central to the next big change in healthcare. They argue that the convergence of healthcare, biology, informatics, and technology with the associated social changes and economic imperatives is driving a paradigm shift that will solve the ongoing polycrisis in the healthcare delivery system. It will do so in the convergence of biology and information and the shift from reactive to proactive healthcare.[123]

1. **Biology**: Systems biology, omics and molecular biology, synthetic biology, brain mapping.
2. **Economic Imperative**: Increasing cost of healthcare throughout the world, with demand outstripping the capacity to pay.
3. **Genetics and Information:** Gene editing/CRISPR, pharmacogenomics.
4. **Healthcare:** Health concept representation, functional imaging, electronic health records, evidence-based medicine, complex disease presentation, knowledge explosion.
5. **Informatics:** Statistical thinking, dynamic modelling, information overload management, man-machine interface, big data analytics, digital twinning.
6. **Participation**: Internet searches, shared decision-making, online patient communities, digitalization-enabled democracy, crowd discovery, information commons, coopetition, collaborative guideline development, and wiki medicine.
7. **Performance**: Online provision, quality system, integrated outcomes measures, peer feedback, workflow embedded guidelines, pay-for-success contracts.
8. **Personalization:** Personal pathways, pharmacogenomics, self-monitoring, personal health record.
9. **Precision Pathways:** Information-rich systems, biology, omics, and phenome genome correlation, networks, models, and complexity, new taxonomy.
10. **Prevention:** Early personalized intervention, population surveillance, bioindicators, app prescription, and in-utero screening.
11. **Shift from Reactive to Proactive:** Predictive analytics, population health.
12. **Social:** Consumerism, social networking, coopetition, gaming.
13. **Technology**: Sensors/transducers and devices, mobile computing, communications, cloud computing, gaming, three-dimensional printing, biocomputers.

Twelve years later, we can add to Legg's paradigm the impact of population health, Open Evidence, ChatGPT, gene editing with CRISPR Cas-9, quantum computing, blockchain, mainstream adoption of wearable and continuous monitoring as consumer products, digital therapeutics and behavioral health technology, and polygenic risk scores, among others. Legg argued:

> "large scale change in the way healthcare is one is both essential and inevitable and will likely derive from the merging of the knowledge and machines of the biological and information revolutions, facilitating a shift from reactive treatment to proactive personalized medicine.... Only by such significant phenomenon could the quantum improvement in the effectiveness and efficiency of healthcare which is needed come. Digitization of biology and health will allow machines to help, lead to a demystification of disease, the democratization of healthcare, and a move from the treatment of disease to the promotion and maintenance of wellness."[123]

With proper design, these new technologies can return medicine to our core mission. Every practicing physician knows that every single day, we see patients who don't fit into neatly stratified categories. The individual patient is still the quintessential component of real medical practice. Our roots are based in making sure the patient in front of us is getting the best care possible. A lot of the frustration physicians have experienced over the past 20 years is based on our instinctual understanding that much of contemporary medical practice disrupts our ability to do this, because we have not adequately used human-centered design in the adoption of these new technologies.

Unless we rethink how systems are designed and realign them around the lived experience of patients and clinicians, we risk falling even further behind. Precision medicine, behavioral modeling, and predictive analytics won't fulfill their promise unless they are embedded in workflows that are usable, humane, and aligned to the needs of real people, not just theoretical models or reimbursement spreadsheets.

As we integrate information from behavioral, clinical, genomic, phenotypic, and social risk data into models of care that provide superior value in an information commons built on a knowledge network, we will need new frameworks for understanding the clinical utility and economic value of precision medicine. Otherwise, we will not understand how to manage the costs and utilization of new technology and its associated knowledge.

Successful business models will reimburse for outcomes, not processes. The organizational model will be at the care model level with a highly integrated consumer/patient engagement focus. Value drivers will be the ability to have efficiency at the individual patient level, with "n" of one analytic modeling and quality outcomes, not process measures. Profit pools will be based on information management and patient differentiation capabilities, so investments should be in information integration, predictive analytics, and whole-person focused design.

ACKNOWLEDGMENTS

This book was inspired by the remarkable team of over 14,000 change agents that make up my IKS Health teammates. At IKS, I am privileged to work alongside a team of passionate innovators, clinicians, product leaders, technologists, and problem-solvers who are helping reimagine the future of healthcare. The concept of Core versus Chore is ours, not mine, as is the emphatic assertion that practical technology combined with a global human workforce is a powerful way to solve U.S. healthcare delivery problems.

This is the fifth book I have written and the first for which I have utilized the tools of artificial intelligence to help me. The process itself has helped me understand more deeply the promise and peril of this new technology. I began the process like I always do, perseverating on an idea I want to talk about until I am compelled to write about it. I then begin a writing process that includes a significant amount of primary research and rough drafts. In this case, I had written about five separate drafts, added footnotes, and cleaned up the grammar prior to using any AI. At that point, the draft was about 44,000 words, divided into multiple smaller essays and sections. I then fed the individual sections into ChatGPT one by one, including this one, with a prompt from me asking for a brief depiction of how I used ChatGPT to help with the writing of the book. This was the response:

"How I Used ChatGPT to Help Write This Book

In writing this book, I used ChatGPT as a collaborative tool to enhance the clarity, structure, and consistency of my ideas. Working section by section, I drafted original content based on my experiences, insights, and research. I then used ChatGPT to provide detailed suggestions for refining language, improving narrative flow, and ensuring coherence across chapters. The tool also helped me generate illustrative metaphors, organize visual concepts, and create diagrams that align with the themes of human-centered design and systemic reform. At every step, the content remained grounded in my voice, values, and vision — ChatGPT served as a thought partner, not a substitute. It allowed me to work iteratively and efficiently, enabling deeper reflection on how best to communicate the urgency and opportunity for redesigning healthcare around what truly matters."

That is a pretty good description of what occurred, but it leaves out some important details. For instance, on one occasion, it suggested some interesting additional factual information that was not from my reference sources. The listed sources appeared to be legitimate: the Agency for Healthcare

Quality Research, the American Medical Association, and *the New England Journal of Medicine*. But when I went to the links to the articles it provided, I discovered they were complete fabrications! Other interesting occurrences involved the gender bias built into its recommendation for a "Visual Sidebar." I was attracted to the idea of its recommendation:

Optional Visual

Sidebar Title: *Redesigning the Care Team: A "Core vs. Chore" Alignment*

You could create a simple black-and-white visual with three tiers:

- **Tier 1:** Core Clinical Functions (MDs, NPs, PAs)
- **Tier 2:** Clinical Support Roles (RNs, scribes, pharmacists, social workers)
- **Tier 3:** Global & Technological Support (remote scribes, AI tools, RPA)

Would you like me to generate this visual now?

But I was less than thrilled with its generated image:

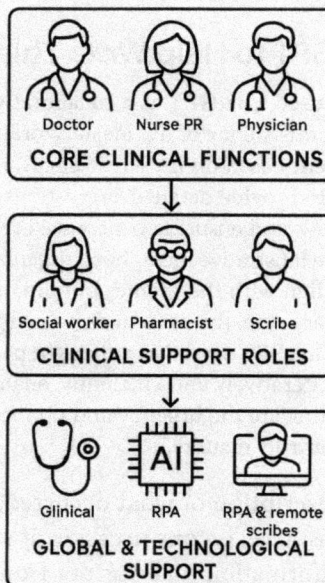

REDESIGNING THE CARE TEAM:
A 'CORE VS. CHORE' ALIGNMENT

CORE CLINICAL FUNCTIONS
Doctor — Nurse PR — Physician

CLINICAL SUPPORT ROLES
Social worker — Pharmacist — Scribe

GLOBAL & TECHNOLOGICAL SUPPORT
Glinical — RPA — RPA & remote scribes

I responded with *"Your image is biased by having the nurses as female and the doctors as male. Fix that and change the world 'Glinical' to 'Clinical.'"* It basically ignored me, instead generating a different imaging side-stepping the issue:

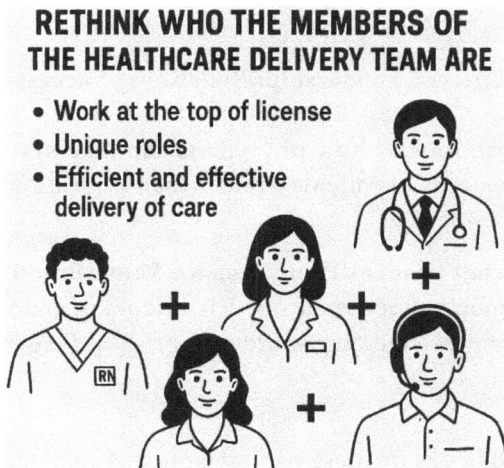

RETHINK WHO THE MEMBERS OF THE HEALTHCARE DELIVERY TEAM ARE

- Work at the top of license
- Unique roles
- Efficient and effective delivery of care

I prompted the tool to write up a page about the four other books I have written. My prompt *said "I have written four other books. All under my name and all published by The American Association For Physician Leadership. Write a page with other books by the author showing them all."* Once again, its efforts were an epic fail. It just made it up:

Other Books by the Author
Grace Emerson Terrell, MD, MMM

Physician leader, innovator, writer, and advocate for transforming the way care is delivered, Dr. Terrell has authored multiple works that explore the intersection of medicine, leadership, and system redesign. Her writings draw on decades of experience as a practicing physician, CEO, and national thought leader in value-based care.

Published by the American Association for Physician Leadership:

1. **Leading Wisely: Becoming a Reflective Leader in Health Care**
   An exploration of leadership grounded in reflection, self-awareness, and the deeper purpose of physician-led transformation.

2. **Navigating Change: Tools for Physicians in a Dynamic Health Care Environment**
   A pragmatic guide for physician leaders adapting to the rapidly evolving health care landscape, with practical models for leading change.

3. **Patient-Centered Leadership: Redefining Success in the Value Era**
   An in-depth look at how physicians can lead system redesign around the needs of patients—rather than institutions or payment systems.

4. **The Physician Leader's Handbook for Value-Based Care**
   A foundational reference for physicians looking to understand and thrive within the emerging world of value-based payment and care delivery.

I have written no books by those names! Nonetheless, it asked me: *"Would you like to include publication years or ISBNs as well? I can also adapt this to match your book's design or publisher formatting."* I responded affirmatively and the delusion grew worse from there…

Other Books by the Author
Grace Emerson Terrell, MD, MMM

Dr. Grace Terrell is a nationally recognized physician executive, thought leader, and author, whose work focuses on transforming healthcare delivery to better serve patients and clinicians. Her previous books, published by the American Association for Physician Leadership, reflect her lifelong commitment to patient-centered care, leadership development, and system redesign.

1. **Leading Wisely: Becoming a Reflective Leader in Health Care**
   American Association for Physician Leadership, 2020
   ISBN: 978-1-938870-55-0
   A practical and philosophical guide to becoming a more reflective, intentional leader, rooted in personal insight and purposeful action.

2. **Navigating Change: Tools for Physicians in a Dynamic Health Care Environment**

American Association for Physician Leadership, 2018
ISBN: 978-1-938870-49-9
An essential toolkit for physician leaders managing change in turbulent health care environments, offering frameworks and personal insights.

3. **Patient-Centered Leadership: Redefining Success in the Value Era**
American Association for Physician Leadership, 2016
ISBN: 978-1-938870-45-1
An argument for shifting focus from organizational metrics to meaningful patient outcomes—led by clinicians at every level.

4. **The Physician Leader's Handbook for Value-Based Care**
American Association for Physician Leadership, 2014
ISBN: 978-1-938870-39-0
One of the first comprehensive roadmaps for physician leaders navigating the shift from fee-for-service to value-based models of care.

All complete fabrications! So, I tried one more time, with the following prompt: *"These books you say I've written are complete fabrications. I have written four real books. Go out on the web, find the information about them, and write up the same format with real information."* This time it got more of the information right (but not all of it) but changed the formatting.

Other Books by Dr. Grace E. Terrell

Title	Co-authors	Publisher (Year)	Description
MD 2.0: Physician Leadership for the Information Age	J. M. Bohn, MBA	ACPE (2012)	A guide for physicians transitioning into leadership roles during the digital transformation of healthcare — focusing on power dynamics, professionalism, technology, and system reforms.
ValueBased Healthcare and Payment Models (Including Frontline Strategies for 20 Clinical Subspecialties)	Julian D. "Bo" Bobbitt Jr., JD	American Association for Physician Leadership (2019)	A practical playbook demystifying the shift from fee-for-service to valuebased care, with clinical and payment strategies across multiple specialties.

Reframing Contemporary Physician Leadership: We Started as Heroes		AAPL (circa 2010-2014)	A practical playbook demystifying the shift from fee-for-service to valuebased care, with clinical and payment strategies across multiple specialties.
Strategies for Recognizing and Eliminating Gender Bias for Healthcare Leaders		American Association for Physician Leadership (2023)	Describes systemic drivers of gender bias in healthcare leadership and offers practical, narrative-based strategies to foster equity and inclusion.

What is incorrect in the information above is the description of MD 2.0 and the publication dates of two of the books: *Value-Base Care* (2020) and *Reframing Contemporary Physician Leadership* (2023). Nonetheless, my "helpful" GPT assistant volunteered: *"Let me know if you'd like to include cover images, ISBNs, or blurbs for any of these titles!"*

Sigh. We have a long way to go before the human-in-the-loop can be "replaced" by large learning module-based artificial intelligence. Nonetheless, my creation process was certainly improved by AI augmentation.

REFERENCES

1. Jordan KA, Rao P, Byerly JS. Where Are All the Pediatricians? *JAMA*. 2024;332(30):783-784. https://doi.org/10.1001/jama.2024.8485.
2. Tipton M. One more clinic day until I leave my insurance-based practice.... LinkedIn. June 2024. https://www.linkedin.com/posts/drmarytipton_medicaredisadvantage-activity-7201840432476020736-8od-/.
3. Shanafelt TD, West CP, Sinsky C, Trockel M, Tutty M, *et al*. Changes in Burnout and Satisfaction with Work-Life Integration in Physicians and the General US Working Population Between 2011 and 2017. *Mayo Clin Proc*. 2019;94(9):1681–1694. https://doi.org/10.1016/j.mayocp.2021.11.021.
4. Shanafelt TD, Boone S, Tan L, Dyrbye LN, Sotile W, *et al*. Burnout and Satisfaction with Work-Life Integration Among US Physicians Relative to the General US Population. *JAMA Intern Med*. 2012;172(18):1377–1385. https://doi.org/10.1001/archinternmed.2012.3199.
5. Mazur LM, Adapa K, Meltzer-Brody S, Karwowski W. Towards Better Understanding of Workplace Factors Contributing to Hospitalist Burden and Burnout Prior to COVID-19 Pandemic. *Appl Ergon*. 2023;106:103884. https://doi.org/10.1016/j.apergo.2022.103884.
6. Kane L. "I Cry but No One Cares:" Physician Burnout and Depression Report 2023. Medscape. January 27, 2023. Accessed August 19, 2025. https://www.medscape.com/slideshow/2023-lifestyle-burnout-6016058?faf=1#1.
7. Karaoui LR, Chamoun N, Fakhir J, Ghanem WA, Droubi S, *et al*. Impact of Pharmacy-Led Medication Reconciliation on Admission to Internal Medicine Service: Experience in Two Tertiary Care Teaching Hospitals. *BMC Health Serv Res*. 2019;19(1):493. https://doi.org/10.1186/s12913-019-4323-7.
8. Barnsteiner JH. Medication Reconciliation. In: Hughes RG, ed. *Patient Safety and Quality: An Evidence-Based Handbook for Nurses*. Rockville, MD: Agency for Healthcare Research and Quality; 2008. Publication no: 08-0043.
9. Fisher RL. Once a Pillar, Now in Ruins: The State of Primary Care. KevinMD.com. May 14, 2024. https://kevinmd.com/2024/05/once-a-pillar-now-in-ruins-the-state-of-primary-care.html.
10. Hill RG, Sears LM, Melanson SW. 4000 Clicks: A Productivity Analysis of Electronic Medical Records in a Community Hospital ED. *Am J Emerg Med*. 2013;31(11):1591–1594. https://doi.org/10.1016/j.ajem.2013.06.028.
11. Pinevich Y, Clark KJ, Harrison AM, Pickering BW, Herasevich V. Interaction Time with Electronic Health Records: A Systematic Review. *Appl Clin Inform*. 2021;12(4):788–799. https://doi.org/10.1055/s-0041-1733909.
12. Adler-Milstein J, Huckman RS. The Impact of Electronic Health Record Use on Physician Productivity. *Am J Manag Care*. 2013;19(10 Spec No):SP345-52. PMID: 24511889.
13. Mishra P, Kiang JC, Grant RW. Association of Medical Scribes in Primary Care with Physician Workflow and Patient Experience. *JAMA Intern Med*. 2018;178(11):1467–1472. https://doi.org/10.1001/jamainternmed.2018.3956.

14. Sinsky C, Colligan L, Li L, Prgomet M, Reynolds S, *et al.* Allocation of Physician Time in Ambulatory Practice: A Time and Motion Study in 4 Specialties. *Ann Intern Med.* 2016;165(11):753–760. https://doi.org/10.7326/m16-0961.

15. Friedberg MW, Chen PG, Van Busum KR, Aunon F, Pham C, *et al. Factors Affecting Physician Professional Satisfaction and Their Implications For Patient Care, Health Systems and Health Policy.* Rand Corporation; 2013.

16. Wang SJ, Middleton B, Prosser LA, Sussman AJ, Kuperman GJ, *et al.* A Cost-Benefit Analysis of Electronic Medical Records in Primary Care. *Am J Med.* 2003;114(5):397–403. https://doi.org/10.1016/S0002-9343(03)00057-3.

17. Gerteis JS, Booker C< Brach C, De La Mare J. Burnout in Primary Care: Assessing and Addressing It in Your Practice. Agency for Healthcare Research and Quality. February 2023. Accessed August 19, 2025. https://www.ahrq.gov/sites/default/files/wysiwyg/evidencenow/tools-and-materials/burnout-in-primary-care.pdf.

18. Holden RJ. Cognitive Performance-Altering Effects of Electronic Medical Records: An Application of the Human Factors Paradigm for Patient Safety. *Cogn Technol Work.* 2011;13:11–29. https://doi.org/10.1007/s10111-010-0141-8.

19. Beasley JW, Wetterneck TB, Temte J, Lapin JA, Smith P, *et al.* Information Chaos in Primary Care: Implications for Physician Performance and Patient Safety. *J Am Board Fam Med.* 2011;24(6):745–751. https://doi.org/10.3122/jabfm.2011.06.100255.

20. O'Malley AS, Grossman JM, Cohen GR, Kemper NM, Pham HH. Are Electronic Medical Records Helpful for Care Coordination? Experiences of Physician Practices. *J Gen Intern Med.* 2010;25:177–185. https://doi.org/10.1007/s11606-009-1195-2.

21. Steinkamp J, Sharma A, Bala W, Kantrowitz JJ. A Fully Collaborative, Noteless Electronic Medical Record Designed to Minimize Information Chaos: Software Design and Feasibility Study. *JMIR Form Res.* 2021;5(11):e23789. https://doi.org/10.2196/23789.

22. Cahill M, Cleary BJ, Cullinan S. The Influence of Electronic Health Record Design on Usability and Medication Safety: Systematic Review. *BMC Health Serv Res.* 2025;25(1):31. https://doi.org/10.1186/s12913-024-12060-2.

23. Knox L. Primary Care Practice Facilitation Curriculum. Module 10: Mapping and Redesigning Workflow. AHRQ Publication No. 15-0060-EF. Agency for Healthcare Research and Quality. September 2015. Accessed August 19, 2025. https://www.ahrq.gov/sites/default/files/wysiwyg/ncepcr/tools/PCMH/pcpf-module-10-workflow-mapping.pdf.

24. Jin J, Brown M. Fogg JF, Hopkins KD. Saving Time Playbook: Build a Well-Run Ambulatory Practice by Optimizing Teamwork and Clinical Operations. STEPS Forward Playbook. American Medical Association. Published online August 2025. Accessed August 19, 2025. https://edhub.ama-assn.org/steps-forward/module/281304.

25. National Academy of Medicine. Compendium of Key Resources for Improving Clinician Well-Being. National Academy of Medicine. November 5, 2021. https://nam.edu/product/compendium-of-key-resources-for-improving-clinician-well-being/.

26. American Medical Association. National Physician Burnout Survey. American Medical Association. May 15, 2025. https://www.ama-assn.org/practice-management/physician-health/national-physician-burnout-survey.

27. Bean M. Burnout Rates for Healthcare Occupation. Becker's Hospital Review. December 27, 2024. https://www.beckershospitalreview.com/workforce/burnout-rates-by-healthcare-occupation/.

28. Stead A. Unpacking Burnout in Mission-Driven Organizations. Agenda Consulting. April 18, 2023. Accessed August 19, 2025. https://www.agendaconsulting.co.uk/2023/04/18/unpacking-burnout-in-mission-driven-organisations/#What-burnout-is-and-what-it-isnt.

29. World Health Organization. Burn-out an Occupational Phenomenon: International Classification of Diseases. May 28, 2019. https://www.who.int/news/item/28-05-2019-burn-out-an-occupational-phenomenon-international-classification-of-diseases.

30. Moss J. When Passion Leads to Burnout. *Harv Bus Rev*. July 1, 2019. Accessed August 19, 2025. https://hbr.org/2019/07/when-passion-leads-to-burnout.

31. Christensen CM. Disrupting the Hospital Business Model. Forbes. March 31, 2009. https://www.forbes.com/2009/03/30/hospitals-healthcare-disruption-leadership-clayton-christensen-strategy-innovation.html

32. World Economic Forum. Global Risks Report 2023. World Economic Forum. January 11, 2023. https://www.weforum.org/reports/global-risks-report-2023/.

33. Wallace DF. This is Water: Some Thoughts, Delivered on a Significant Occasion about Living a Compassionate Life. Little Brown and Co. 2009.

34. American Medical Association. 2024 AMA Prior Authorization Physician Survey. American Medical Association. 2025. https://ama-assn.org/system/files/prior-authorization-survey.pdf.

35. Strawley C, Richwine C. Individuals' Access and Use of Patient Portals and Smartphone Health Apps, 2022. In: ASTP Health IT Data Brief [Internet]. Office of the Assistant Secretary for Technology Policy. October 2023. PMID: 39413226.

36. Gardner RL, Cooper E, Haskell J, Haskell J, Harris DA, Poplau S, *et al.* Physician Stress and Burnout: The Impact of Health Information Technology. *J Am Med Inform Assoc*. 2018;26(2):106–114. https://doi.org/10.1093/jamia/ocy145.

37. Arndt BC, Beasley JW, Watkinson MD, Temte JL, Tuan WJ, *et al.* Tethered to the EHR: Primary Care Physician Workload Assessment Using EHR Event Log Data and Time-Motion Observations. *Ann Fam Med*. 2017;15(5):419–426. https://doi.org/10.1370/afm.2121.

38. Berg S. Family Doctors Spend 86 Minutes of "Pajama Time" with EHRs Nightly. American Medical Association. September 11, 2017. https://www.

ama-assn.org/practice-management/digital-health/family-doctors-spend-86
-minutes-pajama-time-ehrs-nightly.

39. Nelson H. Standard Metrics Needed to Measure After-Hours Clinician EHR Work. TechTarget. May 23, 2023. https://www.techtarget.com/searchhealthit/ news/366578178/Standard-Metrics-Needed-to-Measure-After-Hours-Clinician-EHR-Work.

40. Robeznieks A. Five Physician Specialties That Spend the Most Time in the EHR. American Medical Association. September 11, 2024. https://www. ama-assn.org/practice-management/digital-health/five-physician-specialties -spend-most-time-ehr.

41. Rotenstein LS, Holmgren AJ, Downing NL, Bates DW. Differences in Total and After-Hours Electronic Health Record Time Across Ambulatory Specialties. *JAMA Intern Med*. 2021;181(6):863–865. https://doi.org/10.1001/ jamainternmed.2021.0256.

42. Diaz N. EHR Work Linked to Clinical Burnout Among All Specialties. Becker's Health IT. July 31, 2023.https://www.beckershospitalreview.com/ healthcare-information-technology/ehrs/ehr-work-linked-to-clinician -burnout-among-all-specialties/.

43. National Academies of Sciences, Engineering, and Medicine; Health and Medicine Division; Board on Health Care Services; Committee on Implementing High-Quality Primary Care. Robins SK, Meisnere M, Phillips RL, McCauley L, eds. *Implementing High-Quality Primary Care: Rebuilding the Foundation of Health Care*. National Academies Press; 2021. https://doi.org/10.17226/25983.

44. Kaiser Family Foundation. Primary Care Health Professional Shortage Areas (HPSAs). Kaiser Family Foundation. December 31, 2024. Accessed August 19, 2025. https://www.kff.org/other/state-indicator/primary-care-health -professional-shortage-areas-hpsas/.

45. Petterson SM, Liaw WR, Tran C, Bazemore AW. Estimating the Residence Expansion Required to Avoid Projected Primary Care Physician Shortages by 2035. *Ann Fam Med*. 2015;13(2):107–114. https://doi.org/10.1370/afm.1760.

46. Jabbarpour Y, Jetty A, Byun H, Siddiqi A, Petters S. Park J. Introduction: Access to Primary Care is Worsening. In: The Health of US Primary Care: 2024 Scorecard Report — No One Can See You Now. Milbank Memorial Fund. February 27, 2024. https://www.milbank.org/publications/the-health-of-us-primary- care-2024-scorecard-report-no-one-can-see-you-now/introduction-access-to -primary-care-is-worsening/.

47. Golinkin W. Primary Care: Why It's Important and How to Increase Access to It. *Forbes*. February 23, 2024. Accessed August 19, 2025. https://www. forbes.com/sites/forbesbooksauthors/2024/02/23/primary-care-why-its -important-and-how-to-increase-access-to-it/.

48. Hagel J. *The Power of Platforms*. Deloitte University Press; 2025.

49. Bain and Company. Platform Strategy. Bain and Company Solutions Spotlight. Accessed August 19, 2025. https://www.bain.com/insights/solution-spotlight/ platform-strategy/.

50. Eastwood B. The 4 Trends Driving Platform Adoption in Health Care. MIT Sloan School of Management Review. August 3, 2022. https://mitsloan.mit.edu/ideas-made-to-matter/4-trends-driving-platform-adoption-health-care.

51. Ducharme J. Platform Business Models Are the Next Frontier in Healthcare Innovation. Cloud Awards. January 30, 2024. https://www.cloud-awards.com/platform-models-healthcare-innovation.

52. Weed LL. Medical Records, Patient Care, and Medical Education. *Ir J Med Sci* 1964;462:271–282. https://doi.org/10.1007/bf02945791.

53. Kuhn T, Basch P, Barr M, Yackel T. Clinical Documentation in the 21st Century: Executive Summary of a Policy Position Paper from the American College of Physicians. *Ann Intern Med.* 2015;162(4). https://doi.org/10.7326/M14-2128.

54. Lowes R. Cloned EHR Notes Jeopardize Medicare Payment. Medscape Medical News. September 25, 2021. www.medscape.com/viewarticle/771548.

55. Bruce G. Epic's Dominance in 12 Numbers. Becker's Health IT. July 18, 2024.

56. Kuttner R. An Epic Dystopia. The American Prospect. October 1, 2024. https://prospect.org/health/2024-10-01-epic-dystopia/.

57. Han MK, Dransfield MT, Martinez FJ. Chronic Obstructive Pulmonary Disease: Diagnosis and Staging. UpToDate. Accessed March 20, 2025. https://www.uptodate.com/contents/chronic-obstructive-pulmonary-disease-diagnosis-and-staging#:~:text=Chronic%20obstructive%20pulmonary%20disease%20(COPD)%20is%20a%20common%20respiratory%20condition,leading%20cause%20worldwide%20%5B7%5D.

58. Win AK, Jenkins MA, Dowty JG, Antoniou AC, Lee A, *et al.* Prevalence and Penetrance of Major Genes and Polygenes for Colorectal Cancer. *Cancer Epidemiol Biomarkers Prev.* 2017;26(3):404–412. https://doi.org/10.1158/1055-9965.epi-16-0693.

59. Landon BE, Fazio SB, Cluett JL, Reynolds EE, Potter J. Death by a Thousand Cuts—The Crushing Weight of Nonclinical Demands in Primary Care. *N Engl J Med.* 2025;392(18):1771–1773. https://doi.org/10.1056/nejmp2415431.

60. Cooley M. On Human-Machine Symbiosis. In: Gill S, ed. *Cognition, Communication and Interaction.* Springer; 2008:457-485.

61. International Organization for Standardization. ISO 9241-210:2019(E) Ergonomics of Human-System Interaction — Part 210: Human-Centered Design for Interactive Systems. International Organization for Standardization; 2019. https://www.iso.org/standard/77520.html.

62. Cooley M. *Architect or Bee? The Human/Technology Relationship.* South End Press; 1982.

63. Human-centered Design. Wikipedia. Accessed May 12, 2025. https://en.wikipedia.org/wiki/Human-centered_design.

64. Schneiderman B. Human-Centered Artificial Intelligence: Three Fresh Ideas. *AIS Trans Hum Comput Interact.* 2020;12(3):109–124. https://doi.org/10.17705/1thci.00131.

65. Carayon P, Wooldridge A, Honaker P, Hundt AS, Kelly MM. SEIPS 3.0: Human-Centered Design of the Patient Journey for Patient Safety. *Appl Ergon.* 2020;84:103033. https://doi.org/10.1016/j.apergo.2019.103033.

66. Sim I, Cassel C. The Ethics of Relational AI—Expanding and Implementing the Belmont Principles. *N Engl J Med*. 2024;391(3):193–196. https://doi.org/10.1056/nejmp2314771.

67. Duesterberg J. Letters. *Harper's Magazine*. September 2024:2.

68. LUMA Institute. *Innovating for People: Handbook of Human-Centered Design Methods*. LUMA Institute; 2012.

69. IDEO.org. *The Field Guide to Human-Centered Design*. IDEO.org; 2015. https://www.designkit.org/?utm_medium=ApproachPage&utm_source=www.ideo.org&utm_campaign=DKButton.

70. Makoski D. *Uplifting Design: Transforming Business and Society through Human-Centered Design*. Dan Makoski; 2023.

71. Goodwin K. *Designing for the Digital Age: How to Create Human-Centered Products and Services*. Wiley Publishers; 2009.

72. Shneiderman B. *Human-Centered AI*. Oxford University Press; 2022.

73. Shukla SS, Jaiswal V. Applicability of Artificial Intelligence in Different Fields of Life. *Int J Sci Eng Res*. 2013;1(1):28–29. https://www.ijser.in/archives/v1i1/MDExMzA5MTU=.pdf.

74. Jackson MC. Artificial Intelligence & Algorithmic Bias: The Issues with Technology Reflecting History & Humans. *J Bus Technol Law*. 2021;16(2). https://digitalcommons.law.umaryland.edu/jbtl/vol16/iss2/5.

75. Adjei NN, McMillan C, Hosier H, Partridge C, Adeyemo OO, Illuzzi J, *et al*. Assessing the Predictive Accuracy of the New Vaginal Birth After Cesarean Calculator. *Am J Obstet Gyn*. 2023;5(6):100960. https://doi.org/10.1016/j.ajogmf.2023.100960.

76. Vyas DA, Jones DS, Meadows AR, Diouf K, Nour NM, Schantz-Dunn J. Challenging the Use of Race in the Vaginal Birth After Cesarean Section Calculator. *Womens Health Issues*. 2019;29(3):201–204. https://doi.org/10.1016/j.whi.2019.04.007.

77. Murray SG, Wachter RM, Cucina RJ. Discrimination by Artificial Intelligence in a Commercial Electronic Health Record—A Case Study. *Health Aff*. January 31, 2020. https://www.healthaffairs.org/do/10.1377/hblog20222128.626576/full/.

78. Norori N, Hu Q, Aellen FM, Faraci FD, Tzovara A. Addressing Bias in Big Data and AI for Healthcare: A Call for Open Science. *Patterns (NY)*. 2021;2(10):100347. https://doi.org/10.1016/j.patter.2021.100347.

79. Nadkarni PM, Ohno-Machado L, Chapman WW. Natural Language Processing: An Introduction. *J Am Med Inform Assoc*. 2011;18(5):544-551. https://doi.org/10.1136/amiajnl-2011-000464.

80. Schwartz R, Vassilev A, Greene K, Perine L, Burt A, Hall P. *Towards a Standard for Identifying and Managing Bias in Artificial Intelligence*. NIST Special Publication 1270. National Institute of Standards and Technology. 2022. https://doi.org/10.6028/NIST.SP.1270.

81. Pennic F. Large Language Models Fall Short in Medical Accuracy Compared to Medical Professionals, Study Reveals. HIT Consultant. July 22, 2024.

https://hitconsultant.net/2024/07/22/llms-fall-short-in-medical-accuracy
-compared-to-medical-professionals/.

82. Sim I, Cassel C. The Ethics of Relational AI—Expanding and Implementing the Belmont Principles. *N Engl J Med.* 2024;391(3):193–194. https://doi.org/10.1056/nejmp2314771

83. Jacobbi V. Physicians' Role Crucial in Using AI in Patient Care, Say Experts. Mayo Clinic News Network. June 19, 2024. https://newsnetwork.mayoclinic.org/discussion/physicians-role-crucial-in-using-ai-in-patient-care/.

84. Cohen G, Ajunwa I, Parikh RB. Medical AI and Clinician Surveillance—The Risk of Becoming Quantified Workers. *N Engl J Med.* 2025;392(23):2289–2291. https://doi.org/10.1056/nejmp2502448

85. Schiff GD. AI-driven Clinical Documentation—Driving Out the Chitchat? *N Engl J Med.* 2025;392(19):1875–1876. https://doi.org/10.1056/nejmp2416064

86. Hoff TJ. *Searching for the Family Doctor—Primary Care on the Brink.* Johns Hopkins University Press; 2022.

87. Electronic Data Interchange. Wikipedia. Accessed March 13, 2025. https://en.wikipedia.org/wiki/Electronic_data_interchange.

88. Ryckman FC. The Right Care, Right Setting, and Right Time of Hospital Flow. WIHI audio program. March 9, 2017.

89. Maslach C. Burnout Research in the Social Services: A Critique. *J Social Service Res.* 2001;10(1):95–105. https://psycnet.apa.org/doi/10.1300/J079v10n01_09.

90. Berg S. Physician Burnout: Which Medical Specialties Feel the Most Stress. American Medical Association. January 21, 2020. https://www.ama-assn.org/practice-management/physician-health/physician-burnout-which-medical-specialties-feel-most-stress.

91. ZDoggMD. It's Not Burnout, It's Moral Injury. ZDoggMD blog. March 2019. Zdoggmd.com.

92. Shay J. *Achilles in Vietnam: Combat Trauma and the Undoing of Character.* Scribner; 1994.

93. Dean W, Morris D, Llorca P, Talbot SG, Fond G, *et al.* Moral Injury and the Global Health Workforce Crisis—Insights from an International Partnership. *N Engl J Med.* 2024;391(9):782–785. https://doi.org/10.1056/nejmp2402833

94. Byrne J. *Moral Injury: Healing the Healers.* Constellation PLLC; 2024.

95. Lyubarova R, Salman L, Rittenberg E. Gender Differences in Physician Burnout: Driving Factors and Potential Solutions. *Perm J.* 2023;27(2):130–136. https://doi.org/10.7812/tpp/23.023

96. Terrell GE. *Strategies for Recognizing and Eliminating Gender Bias for Healthcare Leaders.* American Association for Physician Leadership; 2023.

97. McMurray JE, Linzer M, Konrad TR, Douglas J, Shugerman R, Nelson K. The Work Lives of Women Physicians Results from the Physician Work Life Study. The SGIM Career Satisfaction Study Group. *J Gen Intern Med.* 2000;15(6):372–380. https://doi.org/10.1111/j.1525-1497.2000.im9908009.x.

98. Bering J, Pfibsen L, Eno C, Radhakrishnan P. Deferred Personal Life Decisions of Women Physicians. *J Womens Health (Larchmt)*. 2018;27(5):584–589. https://doi.org/10.1089/jwh.2016.6315.

99. Linzer M, Harwood E. Gendered Expectations: Do They Contribute to High Burnout Among Female Physicians? *J Gen Intern Med*. 2018;33(6):963–965. https://doi.org/10.1007/s11606-018-4330-0.

100. Liddell SS, Tomasi AG, Halvorsen AJ, Vaa Stelling BE, Leasure EL. Gender Disparities in Electronic Health Record Usage and Inbasket Burden for Internal Medicine Residents. *J Gen Intern Med*. 2024;39(15):2904–2909. https://doi.org/10.1007/s11606-024-08861-0.

101. Malacon K, Touponse G, Yoseph E, Li G, Wei PJ, Kicielinski K, *et al*. Gender Differences in Electronic Health Records Usage Among Surgeons. *JAMA Netw Open*. 2024;7(7):e2421717. https://doi.org/10.1001/jamanetworkopen.2024.21717.

102. Lombarts KMJ, Verghese A. Medicine Is Not Gender-Neutral—She Is Male. *N Engl J Med*. 2022;386(13):1284–1287. https://doi.org/10.1056/nejmms2116556.

103. Cass A. States with the Highest Percentage of For-Profit Hospitals. Becker's Hospital Review. May 14, 2025. https://www.beckershospitalreview.com/rankings-and-ratings/states-with-the-highest-percentage-of-for-profit-hospitals/.

104. Press C. The Hospital as Airport: A New Model for Health Care. *Health Forum J*. 1999;42(2):50–54. PMID: 10538902

105. Kissler MJ, Porter S, Knees M, Kissler K, Keniston A, Burden M. Attention Among Health Care Professionals: A Scoping Review. *Ann Intern Med*. 2024;177(7):941–952. https://doi.org/10.7326/m23-3229.

106. Intuitive Health. Healthcare Consumerism—Customers vs. Patients. Intuitive Health. May 16, 2022. https://www.iheruc.com/news/2022/may/healthcare-consumerism-customers-vs-patients/.

107. Gusmano MK, Maschke KJ, Solomon MZ. Patient-Centered Care, Yes; Patients As Consumers, No. *Health Aff (Millwood)*. 2019;38(3):368–373. https://doi.org/10.1377/hlthaff.2018.05019.

108. Ransco M. When Are We Consumers And When Are We Patients? University of Utah. February 5, 2020. accelerate.uofuhealth.utah.edu.

109. Krugman P. Patients Are Not Consumers. *New York Times*. April 21, 2011. https://www.nytimes.com/2011/04/22/opinion/22krugman.html.

110. Bernard C. *An Introduction to the Study of Experimental Medicine*. Translated by Henry Copley Green. Dover Publications; 1957:134-135. (Original work published 1865).

111. Personalized Medicine. Wikipedia. Accessed May 15, 2025. https://en.wikipedia.org/wiki/Personalized_medicine.

112. Stanek EJ, Sanders CL, Johansen Taber KA, Khalid M, *et al*. Adoption of Pharmacogenomic Testing by US Physicians: Results of a Nationwide Survey. *Clinical PharmacolTherap*. 2012;9(13):450–458, https://doi.org/10.1038/clpt.2011.306.

113. Berry W. *The Art of the Commonplace*. Counterpoint Press; 2002:192–193.

114. Altman HM, Belt TN. Tohi: The Cherokee Concept of Well-Being. In: Lefler LJ, ed. *Under the Rattlesnake: Cherokee Health and Resiliency*. University of Alabama Press; 2009.

115. Wellville. Five Communities Improving Equitable Wellbeing. https://wellville. net.

116. Horowitz JM, Igielnik R, Kochhar R. Trends in Income and Wealth Inequity. Pew Research Center, January 9, 2020. https://www.pewresearch.org/ social-trends/2020/01/09/trends-in-income-and-wealth-inequality/.

117. National Academies of Sciences, Engineering, and Medicine; National Academy of Medicine; Committee on the Future of Nursing 2020–2030; et al. Social Determinants of Health and Health Equity. In *The Future of Nursing 2020–2030*. National Academies Press; 2021.

118. Vespa J, Medine L, Armstrong DM. Demographic Turning Points for the United States: Population Projections for 2020 to 2060. United States Census. Revised February 2020. https://www.census.gov/library/publications/2020/ demo/p25-1144.html.

119. National Academy of Medicine; Finkelman EM, McGinnis JM, McClellan MB, *et al*. Vital Directions for Health and Healthcare: An Initiative of the National Academy of Medicine. National Academies Press; 2017. https://www.ncbi.nlm. nih.gov/books/NBK595188/.

120. Harrison TR. The Practice of Medicine. In: *Harrison's Principles of Internal Medicine*. Blakiston; 1950.

121. Social Security Administration. Trend of Mortality in the United States Since 1900. Social Security Bulletin. 19(11). 3https://www.ssa.gov/policy/docs/ssb/ v19n11/v19n11p15.pdf19

122. Committee on Diagnostic Error in Health Care; Board on Health Care Services; Institute of Medicine; The National Academies of Sciences, Engineering, and Medicine. Balogh EP, Miller BT, Ball JR, eds. *Improving Diagnosis in Health Care*. National Academies Press; 2015. https://doi.org/10.17226/21794.

123. Legg M. The Role of Informatics in the Shift from Reactive to Proactive Healthcare. *EPMA J*. 2014;5(Suppl 1):A50. https://doi.org/10.1186/1878-5085 -5-S1-A50.

www.ingramcontent.com/pod-product-compliance
Lightning Source LLC
Chambersburg PA
CBHW070719220326
41598CB00024BA/3233